Acute Mental Health Nursing

Acute Mental Health Nursing

From Acute Concerns to the Capable Practitioner

Edited by

**Marc Harrison,
David Howard
and
Damian Mitchell**

SAGE Publications
London • Thousand Oaks • New Delhi

Contents

List of Contributors

Ian Baguley qualified as a Mental Health Nurse in 1973 and worked in a range of NHS settings. He started work at University of Manchester 10 years ago and has been involved in developing skills based education courses in areas such as Psychosocial Interventions and Cognitive Behaviour Therapy. He is currently working as National Programme Manager for Mental Health Workforce Development.

Joe Curran is a mental health nurse with experience in acute in-patient, forensic and community settings. He currently has a clinical caseload and is involved in education, training, and some research. His work interests include the application of CBT to in-patient environments, practice-based evidence, and behaviour analysis.

Mike Doyle is a qualified RMN who has worked in mental health services for 18 years. He is currently undertaking Post-Doctoral Research at the University of Manchester and also has a Clinical Advisor role in the North West Adult Forensic Mental Health Service that includes work as a specialist therapist in Psychosocial Interventions.

David Duffy is a Nurse Consultant specialising in suicide and self-harm, currently employed by Bolton, Salford and Trafford Mental Health NHS Trust. David has a Doctoral thesis on the subject of suicidality, and from 2001 was lead co-ordinator of the National Suicide Prevention Strategy for England. With Dr Tony Ryan, he is editor of *New Approaches to Preventing Suicide: A Manual For Practitioners* (Jessica Kingsley, forthcoming).

Julie Dulson completed her nurse training in 1997, working in a range of inpatient settings mostly acute, but also rehabilitation and high dependency. She currently works for Mersey Care NHS trust as a practice development facilitator working within the acute inpatient wards. She has recently been seconded half time as practice development facilitator for the acute solutions project at Sainsbury's Centre for Mental Health, based within the acute wards in Mersey care NHS trust.

Alison Faulkner is a mental health service user/survivor now working as an independent researcher, trainer and writer. She has over 16 years' experience in social research, including around 5 years specialising in qualitative methods, and is currently working on the evaluation of a crisis service in Leeds. She is owned by a small black and white cat.

Kevin Gournay is a Chartered Psychologist and Registered Nurse. He has been involved in policy research and development in inpatient care for the last 10 years. He is an expert witness on inpatient suicide and has continued clinical work throughout his career, latterly using CBT for psychosis as well pursuing his specialist interest in the treatment of severe anxiety disorders.

Richard Gray is a Lecturer and MRC Fellow in Health Services Research at the Institute of Psychiatry, Kings College, London. He qualified as a mental health nurse in 1993 and in 2001 he was awarded his PhD from the Institute of Psychiatry. He has published over 60 papers and book chapters.

Julie Hall has a background in mental health nursing who is currently employed as Care Pathway Manager and Audit Lead for Lincolnshire Partnership NHS Trust where she has led the successful implementation of integrated care pathways and variance reporting systems. Julie is currently supported by an Economic and Social Research Council research scholarship to evaluate the use of integrated care pathways in mental health services.

Marc Harrison has a background in both community and acute mental health nursing. He is currently Head of Curriculum Development and Quality Assurance for HM Prison Service (England and Wales) and is also Honorary Research Fellow at the Institute of Psychiatry. Prior to this he was Senior Research Fellow at the University of Manchester and Senior Project Officer with the WHO 'Nations for Mental Health Programme'.

David Howard began his mental health career at the age of 17 as a nursing cadet and has worked extensively in areas of mental health practice, research and education. He is currently Director of the MSc in Organisational Leadership in Health and Social Care at the University of Nottingham, although he continues his interests in mental health by means of teaching and clinical work.

Ann Jackson, RMN, BA (Hons.), MA, is Senior Practice Development Fellow with the RCN Institute Mental Health Programme. Ann's clinical background is in acute in-patient nursing. Her main research interests include: feminist and anti-oppressive research methodologies/practice and women's mental health.

Mick James qualified as a mental health nurse in 1984 and has worked in a broad range of clinical settings. As a senior nurse, he had practical experience of implementing the use of HoNOS across a mental health service. Mick has been National HoNOS Advisor at the Royal College of Psychiatrists' Research Unit since 2000 and also continues to work as a senior manager in the NHS.

Julia Jones, BA (Hons.), Ph.D, wrote this chapter whilst Research Fellow with the RCN Institute Mental Health Programme. She has conducted a number of research studies in acute in-patient settings. She is currently a Marie Curie fellow at the University of Verona, Italy.

Damian Mitchell was appointed to the post of Head of Healthcare Training for the Prison Service (England and Wales) in July 2002, a post that moved across to NHSU in March 2004. Damian is also Subject Lead within the School of Interprofessional Health and Social Care, NHSU, for Mental Health, Criminal Justice and Offender Services.

Rachel Perkins is a Consultant Clinical Psychologist and Clinical Director of Adult Mental Health Services at South West London and St. George's Mental Health NHS Trust. She is also a user of mental health services, vice-chair of the Manic Depression Fellowship, a Specialist Advisor at the Health and Social Care Advisory Service and a member of the Disability Rights Commission's Mental Health Action Group.

Julie Repper is Senior Research Fellow at Sheffield University and Lead Research Nurse for Sheffield Care Trust. Her research interests include social inclusion, recovery and user and carer involvement. She is currently exploring best practice in the assessment of carers' needs and has recently published, with Dr Rachel Perkins, a book entitled *Social Inclusion and Recovery: A Model for Mental Health Practice*.

Paul Rogers worked as a clinician in secure services for 14 years prior to commencing his research career. His current research includes suicidal thinking and mental disorders in prisoners, and the examination of predictive tools for criminal reconviction. Paul has published over 50 peer reviewed and professional papers and was the recipient of the Professor Annie Altchul Publication Prize in Mental Health in 2001.

Tony Ryan has worked as Service Development Manager and Senior Research Fellow since 2000, initially at the North West Mental Health Development Centre and now for the Health and Social Care Advisory Service (HASCAS), as well as working at the University of Manchester. Tony has also spent 10 years working in the NHS as a mental health nurse in a variety of roles.

Gail W. Stuart is Dean and a tenured Professor in the College of Nursing, and a Professor in the College of Medicine at the Medical University of South Carolina. She is currently President of the American College of Mental Health Administration and a fellow in the American Academy of Nursing. She is a prolific writer possibly best known in nursing for her textbook: *Principles and Practice of Psychiatric Nursing*, now in its 7th edition.

Martin Ward is an independent mental health nursing consultant and director of MW Professional Development Limited. He has 35 years' experience in mental health care, as a nurse, teacher, researcher, politician and writer. He was formerly Director of Mental Health for the Royal College of Nursing, and has a large portfolio of publications and a history of international teaching and supervision.

Foreword

When I first started my career in nursing during the 1960s, there were something over 130,000 in-patient places for people with mental health problems, largely sited in the large Victorian asylums. We now know that literally tens of thousands of patients spent their lives incarcerated, when there was probably no reason why they should not have lived reasonably productive lives in the community. Visionaries such as Jim Birley, George Brown, John Wing, Julian Leff and others, were the driving forces behind deinstitutionalisation in the UK, a process that has now been paralleled worldwide. Without any doubt, deinstitutionalisation has brought major benefits, and the lives of countless people have been improved because they are now able to receive treatment in their own homes and communities, rather than being banished to a distant 'bin'. However, we also have to admit that deinstitutionalisation and the setting up of community mental health teams have been far from free of problems. It needs to be said that the expectations of community care have not been realised and I believe (and I know this is an unpopular view with many of my colleagues), that when Frank Dobson said in 1997, community care has failed, he was substantially correct. I had the great pleasure of providing Frank Dobson with advice at this time, and I know that he recognised that community care had failed, not because of the shortcomings of the dedicated people who are the doctors, nurses, psychologists, social workers and others working in our mental health services, but because of starvation of necessary funding, which had been a problem for more than 20 years. With a few exceptions across the world (Australia being a notable example), there had been no bridging funding made available to start up community mental health teams and no real investment in training the necessary numbers of mental health staff for this work and providing them with the means to deliver psychosocial interventions and other evidence-based treatments. Another set of reasons for the relative failure of community care is connected with a range of complex issues concerning public acceptance of the mentally ill. As a consequence of society's views of mental illness and of under-resourcing we now have the spectre of what Len Stein (the architect, with his collaborator Marianne Test, of assertive community treatment) called transinstitutionalisation; i.e., housing mentally ill people in prisons rather than in humane residential care settings.

It is within this wider context that this book is being published. Its publication is extremely timely given that we have at last realised that the emphasis on community approaches has led to the neglect of the acute care area. This book is a valuable addition to the growing literature on acute care and should provide great encouragement to the frontline staff in this area. More positively, we are beginning to see some real new financial investment in mental health services and while some say this is too little too late, I am optimistic that this new money will make a real difference. One other development which should lead to improvement is the setting up of the National Institute for Mental Health which has an emphasis on improving standards in a uniform and systematic fashion. Thus, new textbooks, such as this, will provide the means of disseminating up-to-date knowledge to services across the country.

The chapters in this book should provide the reader, who may be an undergraduate or an experienced mental health worker, with current perspectives on a range of important topics. I was particularly pleased to accept the offer of contributing a chapter, as when I saw the chapter outline, what struck me was the emphasis on providing humane mental health care, within the context of a sound evidence base. Now that I have been able to read the whole text, I am even more pleased to see that the chapter focus is on topics that will make a real difference to people's lives. These important issues are: psychosocial interventions, medication management, risk assessment and management, and the use of various assessment methods. While the issues of what constitutes evidence, and how that evidence is obtained, preoccupies many academics, these chapters go to the heart of what is important to patient care, and the reader will obtain an overarching, and practical-based, view of each area. In addition, the chapters on integrated care pathways, the analysis of the UK and US systems, and two excellent chapters which focus on social inclusion and patient perspectives will provide much food for thought.

Finally, I was delighted to see a chapter on observation, which sets forth the view that the observation of the most ill patients in our residential settings should be provided within the context of a therapeutic relationship. By bringing together this range of excellent material the editors have also been able to produce a book which addresses the most thorny problems which face most frontline staff for much of their working day. Most importantly, the reader of this book will be availed of a wide range of information which, if put into practice, will improve the quality of services that we provide to one of the most needy groups in our society.

Kevin Gournay CBE
Institute of Psychiatry, King's College London
March 2003

An introduction to acute mental health care: from acute concerns to the capable practitioner

David Howard

This book was written in response to the demands being made on the reshaped mental health services for acute adult in-patient care. Effective integration of in-patient environments are essential for the delivery of the National Service Framework for Mental Health (DoH, 1999), the fundamental document underpinning the Mental Health Policy Implementation Guide for Adult Acute Inpatient Care Provision (DoH, 2002).

This is in direct contrast to the previous 25 years, however, where the majority of mental health policy in the UK focused on developing community-based services (DoH, 2002). While considerable improvements were made, both in the provision of care in the community and in encouraging innovative practices, this was often at the expense of investment in acute in-patient care, despite substantial demands made upon in-patient services caused by:

- a reduction in the numbers of in-patient beds;
- more challenging symptoms of the patients who were admitted (because community staff supported less severely ill patients within the community);
- an increased number of admissions complicated by drug abuse (Higgins et al., 1999; Watson, 2001).

The NHS Plan (DoH, 2000) took the first step in redressing this imbalance. It pledged the government to investing in developing and improving in-patient mental health services and, in April 2001, this commitment was followed up by making £30 million available for upgrading ward environments. However, it was not just the buildings that had been neglected over the previous 25 years. Staff working within in-patient settings had seen investment diverted into high-profile community-based services while at the same time, they were having to meet increased demands on in-patient services with reduced numbers of available in-patient beds while simultaneously coping with more demanding symptom profiles of patients. This was compounded by an apparent devaluing of in-patient care, inconsistent services arising from local funding agendas and trust re-organisations, difficulties in recruiting and retaining in-patient staff and increased levels of sickness – particularly sickness associated with stressful work environments (Hurst, 2000). Furthermore, numerous reports have identified severe shortcomings in mental health care delivery (NIMHE, 2002) and, in turn, this has resulted in the adoption of 'defensive' working practices, the upshot of which in many areas resulted in a doubling of time senior ward staff spent completing paperwork (Higgins et al., 1999).

So within this context, why would anyone want to work within acute in-patient care? Although the situation described above sounds very negative, it must be remembered that it is precisely because of these circumstances that the attention of policy makers turned to the provision of in-patient care. While changes in mental health legislation has set targets for good practice, the means of achieving these targets relies upon the skills and commitment of practitioners within in-patient services.

The government's (long overdue) intention is to raise the profile of in-patient care and to recognise the specialist knowledge and skills of staff working in this area (DoH, 2002). Indeed, within the context of contemporary service delivery, achieving this intention is not an option. For those working within in-patient areas these factors present a rare opportunity to improve and develop in-patient services for the benefit of all stakeholders. This is therefore an exciting time to be working in this area and this period is likely to be seen as a watershed in care delivery in subsequent years. However, to meet these challenges, and to implement changes safely, requires that practitioners are informed and knowledgeable of contemporary practice. It is to support these staff, by supplying a resource of evidence to enable them to achieve these objectives, that this book was written.

A key report into contemporary mental health in-patient care was that of the Standing Nursing and Midwifery Advisory Committee (1999), *Mental Health Nursing "Addressing Acute Concerns"*. Although this was followed by two major publications – *The Capable Practitioner: A Framework and List of the Practitioner Capabilities Required to Implement the National Service Framework for Mental Health* (SCMH, 2001) and *The Mental Health Policy Implementation Guide* (DoH, 2002) – the majority of their recommendations for changes to practice within in-patient care in adult mental health can be traced to the six core areas originally identified by the SNMAC (1999) report. Consequently, the chapters within this book have been clustered around these areas.

- Assessment
- Involving users and carers

- Care management
- Management of risk
- Cognitive, behavioural and family interventions
- Medication management

Assessment

To begin, Joe Curran and Paul Rogers provide an overview of the purpose and practice of assessment in their chapter 'Acute psychiatric in-patient assessment'. By using a funnelling approach (from Hawkins, 1986) they introduce three levels of assessment beginning at the broad level, where open questions are used to gather information about the patient's background. Using this information as its base, the assessment gradually focuses down to specific questions designed to gain insight into specific issues linked to the patient's presentation.

It is at this point that specific, validated, instruments to record symptoms or indicators are introduced. A selection of empirically tested tools is outlined and the difficulties of obtaining accurate measurements are discussed. Finally, the chapter concludes by examining how the factors identified during the assessment can be incorporated within a plan of care.

Mick James and Damian Mitchell continue the section on assessment in their chapter 'Measuring health and social functioning using HoNOS'. A number of recommended outcome indicators make use of Health of the Nation Outcome Scales (HoNOS) and it is the application of these within an acute in-patient unit that is the focus of this chapter. There are numerous measures of outcome in mental health care and the debate surrounding the effective use of outcome data to inform clinical practice and service evaluation extends well beyond the use of HoNOS. However, the brevity and comprehensive overview of functioning provided by the instrument provides a relatively easy way of embedding outcome evaluation as part-and-parcel of routine clinical practice. The importance of linking outcome measurement with service practices and systems (e.g., care programme approach, clinical governance and audit, risk assessment and risk management) are debated. In addition, it is suggested that HoNOS data can complement more specific health outcome enquiries relating to groups of service users or specific service delivery models.

Involving users and carers

In their chapter 'Social inclusion and acute care' Julie Repper and Rachel Perkins identify concepts of social inclusion and social exclusion and how they apply to acute psychiatric care. In particular, the ramifications of being treated for a mental illness on the patient's employment and relationships are discussed, and tentative strategies to counter these are identified. However, implementing these strategies within an acute ward environment, particularly when trying to maintain the involvement of family and friends, can be very difficult. So, to put this into perspective, the chapter concludes by encouraging staff to develop self-awareness by thinking what the ward environment is like for patients, relatives and friends.

Self-awareness is continued in the following chapter, 'Strategies for surviving acute care', in which Alison Faulkner gives a very candid account of experiences of receiving acute in-patient care. Some very moving examples of less than ideal practices are documented; however, the aim of this chapter is not to dwell on these, but to highlight aspects of good practice and explore how they can be developed. This is essential reading for care providers and will help to develop awareness of local practices. This chapter, while critical of some aspects of in-patient care, is not written in a negative fashion and there is much to be learned from the author's positive attitude and enthusiasm.

Care management

Drawing from experiences in the United Kingdom and the United States of America, Martin Ward and Gail Stuart examine how case management has been used to monitor quality and promote cost-effective care. 'Case management: perspectives of the UK and US systems' describes the components of case management and argues for its inclusion within UK mental health services, particularly to support people with enduring mental illnesses, where it would help to integrate health and social care services. This is followed by discussion of case management in the United States and examples are given of nurses acting as case managers. The low uptake of case management within the United Kingdom is discussed and ways that may lead to greater uptake are also highlighted.

This issue is developed in the next chapter, 'Integrated care pathways: the "acute" context'. Here, the progress of care pathways within the mental health system in the United Kingdom is examined. Julie Hall argues that the introduction of care pathways in mental health is an attempt to counter the fragmented care systems between different care providers to improve the overall quality of mental health services. Care pathways are described, and the link between this approach and their integration into the care management approach in the US is made. This is closely followed by a comparison of the motives of each system; the US system aiming to control costs while the care pathways attempt to ensure research-based evidence reaches clinical practice. And it is this latter point that demonstrates the benefits to users of the service, the professionals working within it and the organisations providing it. Following this discussion, the application of care pathways within an acute in-patient setting is demonstrated using documentation that has kindly been supplied by Dr Karen Moody of the State Hospital, Carstairs, to allow readers to make an in-depth evaluation of the process.

Management of risk

In 'Risk assessment and management in acute mental health care', David Duffy, Mike Doyle and Tony Ryan examine risk from the perspectives of risk of self-harm and risk of violence. During the first part of this chapter, different methods of assessing the risk of self-harm are considered. Predicting who is likely to self-harm is notoriously difficult and the implications of false negative predictions when the patient succeeds in self-harming, and the staffing costs of false positive predictions, are discussed. They continue by examining how patients at risk of self-harm are managed and debate the issues of accurate screening, care versus control and the attitudes of care staff. Developing on the inconsistencies highlighted by SNMAC (1999), this section concludes with a discussion on the use of observation policies.

The second part of this chapter considers assessing the risk of violence. Factors associated with violent episodes are identified and, with this in mind, the importance of a multidisciplinary approach to assessment is justified. Within a therapeutic programme to effectively manage risk of violence, the authors consider the rights of the individual within the context of the rights, health and safety of others. Strategies and resources to help in the management of a potentially violent patient follow.

Julia Jones and Ann Jackson develop on these issues in 'Observation'. In this chapter, observation is defined as a therapeutic activity, as opposed to a means of collecting data. The patients who are most likely to require observing are those likely to self-harm and the chapter quickly focuses on this group. The trouble with observation, though, is that it is very intrusive and this forms the crux of the first part of this chapter where the difficulties of maintaining the dignity of a patient who is being observed are contrasted with those incurred when maintaining their safety.

It is safety issues that underpin the next part of the chapter where implications of the disparity throughout the UK, regarding observation policy, are considered. Great progress to resolve these issues was made with the introduction of the four-category system of observation in the SNMAC (1999) report. However, major inconsistencies remain, as the CRAG/SCOTMEG system that is used throughout Scotland only has three categories of observation. Despite their differences, though, both make similar recommendations regarding good practice guidelines and the preparation and support of staff.

Finally, the chapter contrasts policy with the experiences of nurses giving, and patients receiving, observation and discusses how insight into their experiences might be incorporated into current practice.

Cognitive, behavioural and family interventions

This section begins with 'Cognitive behaviour therapy in in-patient care'. Here Kevin Gournay sets in context the use of cognitive behaviour therapy (CBT) with an historical overview of its use within in-patient areas. Its evolution is contrasted with contemporary practice by demonstrating how many CBT activities are already incorporated within the work of mental health staff. To respond to the SNMAC report, it is shown how, through measurement and experimentation, CBT can be developed as an evidence-based framework for practice. Finally, specific CBT techniques, and their applications within practice, are discussed.

Ian Baguley and Julie Dulson continue this section in their chapter 'Psychosocial interventions'. Underpinning the psychosocial intervention (PSI) framework is the stress vulnerability model (Zubin and Spring, 1977), and this is applied to the stress invoked by admission to an acute in-patient area, particularly one where aggressive behaviour is common. The PSI framework is structured around an ongoing process of assessment, formulation, intervention and evaluation and aims to understand problems from the patient's point of view. Ian and Julie show how PSI can aid early identification of relapse, which, in turn, can trigger the early involvement of supporting services, limiting the extent of the problems. Finally, the chapter ends by describing some methods of assessment and education that can be used in areas of in-patient care.

Medication management

Richard Gray begins the chapter 'Medication management' by observing that staff spend a significant amount of time helping individuals suffering from psychotic illnesses to manage their medication. Unfortunately, once discharged from hospital, many patients do not continue to take their medication reliably, and this often leads to a recurrence of symptoms and re-admission – the 'revolving door syndrome', which can be frustrating for all concerned. To help to address this, practitioners need to be able to provide information to patients regarding the way in which medication works, and to be understanding of the effects of the medication from the patient's perspective.

Initially, the modes of action of different anti-psychotic medications are explained and their use in the treatment of psychosis is justified. However, the beneficial effects of the medication can sometimes be counterbalanced by undesirable side-effects and, in turn, this helps to clarify why many patients choose not to comply with taking medication. Richard continues by considering the implications of these issues, both for the individual and for the mental health services. From this base, the chapter progresses to identify factors that may enhance compliance. These are each examined critically, using empirically based evaluations, and the chapter concludes by identifying how the issues raised within this chapter can be incorporated within clinical practice.

Finally

This book provides a core framework from which to develop practice within acute in-patient areas. The chapters were specifically written to address the issues that were identified by SNMAC (1999) and NIMHE (2002) to enable practitioners to base the care they give on a sound, empirical framework. It is our hope for this book to primarily be used as a resource by practitioners by providing the evidence to support day-to-day practice issues, and to empower practitioners to implement the changes needed to improve care and practice within acute mental health in-patient areas. It can be seen from the information within these chapters that the role of in-patient staff can develop to provide specialist as well as generic services, and practitioners need to look beyond traditional ways of working, and fully utilise the CPA framework to enable continuity of care. This may simply occur by promoting more effective communication with community-based staff. However, staff may also choose to use the information within this book creatively, to justify extending in-patient services by including areas of care such as outreach work and extended day hospital services.

In the wider context, however, this book is an invaluable resource for managers to employ within staff development. We based this book on the structure of the SNMAC (1999) report knowing that this would enable practitioners to develop and meet many of the recommendations for improving practice identified within *The Capable Practitioner* (SCMH, 2001) and, in turn, many of the requirements of the National Occupational Standards for Mental Health (NIMHE, 2003). Thus this book is a contemporary resource to raise the profile of mental health in-patient care, providing an evidence base to support the expert knowledge and professional skills of staff working within this specialist setting.

References

Department of Health (1999) *The National Service Framework for Mental Health.* London: The Stationery Office.

Department of Health (2000) *The NHS Plan.* London: The Stationery Office.

Department of Health (2002) *Mental Health Policy Implementation Guide: Adult Acute Inpatient Care Provision.* London: The Stationery Office.

Hawkins, R.P. (1986) 'Selection of target behaviours' in R.O. Nelson, and S.C. Hayes, (eds), *Conceptual Foundations of Behavioral Assessment.* New York: Guilford Press. pp. 331–85.

Higgins, R., Hurst, K. and Wistow, G. (1999) 'Nursing acute psychiatric patients: a quantitative and qualitative study', *Journal of Advanced Nursing*, 29 (1): 52–63.

Hurst, K. (2000) 'Managing and leading psychiatric nursing: Part 1' *Nursing Management*, 6 (10): 8–13.

National Institute for Mental Health in England (NIMHE) (2002) *Cases for Change*: *Hospital Services.* London: The Stationery Office.

NIMHE (2003) National Occupational Standards for Mental Health: Implementation Guide Final Version. London: The Stationery Office.

Sainsbury Centre for Mental Health (SCMH) (2001) *The Capable Practitioner: A Framework and List of the Practitioner Capabilities Required to Implement the National Service Framework for Mental Health.* London: SCMH.

Standing Nursing and Midwifery Advisory Committee (SNMAC) (1999) *Mental Health Nursing 'Addressing Acute Concerns'.* London: The Stationery Office.

Watson, A. (2001) *Detained: Inspection of Compulsory Mental Health Admissions.* London: The Stationery Office.

Zubin, J. and Spring, B. (1977) 'Vulnerability' – a new view of schizophrenia', *Journal of Abnormal Psychology*, 86: 103–26.

ONE

Acute psychiatric in-patient assessment

Joe Curran and Paul Rogers

Introduction

This chapter provides an overview of the assessment process in acute in-patient settings. Often an overlooked area, assessment is a crucial aspect of care as unidentified need, or an inaccurate assessment, may lead to ineffective interventions which can result in longer admission and a greater economic burden for overstretched services. This chapter then offers general details on the main methods of collecting salient information required within acute settings.

There are a number of models available that propose to help clinicians to identify relevant areas of assessment, such as the Hierarchy of Needs (Maslow, 1954; Mathes, 1981) and the Tidal Model (Barker, 2002). However, their true value remains a focus of ongoing debate due to their reliance on conceptual ideologies. As such, they will not be examined in this chapter. Instead, broader principles of assessment will be explored without relying on models offering assumptive views of the patient. Once this value-free assessment is complete, clinicians may then wish to utilise nursing, psychological, medical or social models of intervention.

Background

Effective skills of assessment are fundamental to the practitioner working within an acute in-patient environment. The *Mental Health Policy Implementation Guide* (DoH, 2002: 11), specifies the importance of

… service user centred assessment of needs and risks … carried out using established methods and procedures for measuring symptoms, risk and social functioning.

In addition, the importance of mental health workers possessing the skills to conduct a comprehensive assessment of mental health problems is among the key competencies identified in *The Capable Practitioner* (SCMH, 2001). In a broader context, the Workforce Action Team (2001) describe work done on a functional map that identifies key purposes of mental health services. Key Area C, in particular, states that practitioners should

> ... work with individuals to assess mental health needs, diagnose mental illness, and plan, implement and review programmes of care in the broader context of their lives. (p. 72)

In summary, a comprehensive assessment is patient focused and is conducted by competent practitioners as a fundamental part of the delivery of mental health services.

Assessment goals

A comprehensive assessment results in:

- a detailed and precise description of the problems the patient is experiencing;
- a clear description of the patient's current symptoms;
- a comprehensive risk assessment;
- a description of the patient's social, occupational and domestic circumstances;
- the support available to the patient;
- family/carer perspectives;
- an overall management care plan;
- a treatment care plan;
- methods of evaluation.

The role of the assessor

The assessment of in-patients involves a number of mental health professionals. In some instances each profession generates its own reports independently, storing these in their own sections within the patient's case-notes. In other circumstances a single assessment process may be conducted, where all involved in the patient's care share the same assessment and recording procedures. Whichever method is adopted, clear communication of the findings, and of the subsequent plan, of care is essential.

Figure 1.1   The funnelling approach to assessment (based on Hawkins, 1986)

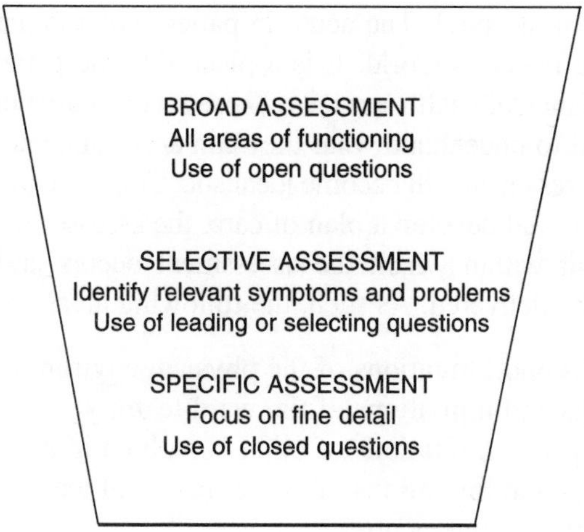

BROAD ASSESSMENT
All areas of functioning
Use of open questions

SELECTIVE ASSESSMENT
Identify relevant symptoms and problems
Use of leading or selecting questions

SPECIFIC ASSESSMENT
Focus on fine detail
Use of closed questions

Assessment framework

> I keep six honest serving men
> (They taught me all I know):
> Their names are What and Why and When,
> And How and Where and Who.

(Rudyard Kipling, 1865–1936)

Hawkins (1986) developed an approach to assessment that is described as 'funnelling' (Figure 1.1). Here, the clinician begins the assessment, taking a broad view of the person and their experiences by assessing a wide variety of areas (e.g., 'What problems does the patient have? Where do these problems occur? When do they occur? With whom do they occur?'). Open-ended questions are used to gather a wide range of information, which on the surface may seem irrelevant; however, it ensures that the assessor is as little influenced as possible by their own, or others', preconceptions about the patient. Funnelling thereafter occurs to identify the fine detail of the problems (e.g., 'When is the problem worse or better?'). Once this has been achieved a complete understanding of the patient's problem can be written as problem statements which become the focus of subsequent treatment or interventions.

The fundamental principle underlying any assessment has the patient and their current experiences at its core. However, a purely symptomatic approach to assessment will not include important contextual factors that may influence the patient's functioning. For this reason it is necessary to assess and understand the nature of the patient's environment prior to (and after) hospitalisation, and to consider the resources available to the patient whilst they are in hospital. The acute in-patient environment is not representative of the patient's world. It is a place that the patient goes for the convenience of mental health services. These services are not perfect, therefore it is crucial to understand what they can and cannot achieve within it, otherwise the assessment will become idealistic. Consequently, to fully assess a patient's needs and develop a plan of care, the assessor needs to consider the environment within which the assessment occurs and within which treatment will be delivered. As such, the following areas are of relevance:

- the strengths and limitations of the physical environment;
- the strengths and limitations of the ward team;
- the strengths and limitations of others involved in the patient's care;
- the strengths and limitations of home treatment teams;
- joint working arrangements;
- ward atmosphere;
- resources;
- discharge arrangements.

What to assess

The English *National Service Framework for Mental Health* (DoH, 1999: 22) notes:

> Assessment should cover psychiatric, psychological and social functioning, risk to the individual and others, including previous violence and criminal record, any needs arising from co-morbidity, and personal circumstances including family or other carers, housing, financial and occupational status.

Assessing symptoms

A broad-based approach to assessment comes from the bio-psycho-social perspective that incorporates biological, psychological and social aspects of a person's experience. For example: biological (e.g., physical functioning, diet, physical investigations and sleep); psychological (e.g., mood, thoughts, feeling states, behaviour, affect, early warning signs for symptoms and relapse indicators/signatures); and social (e.g., social support, family situation, housing, occupation and spirituality).

Assessing risk

Again, the *National Service Framework for Mental Health* (DoH, 1999: 22) notes:

Evidence suggests that the quality of the initial assessments is enhanced when it is multi-disciplinary and undertaken in partnership between health and social care staff. All staff involved in performing assessments should receive training in risk assessment and risk management, updated regularly. A locally agreed pro-forma should be used, with all decisions recorded and communicated to colleagues on a need to know basis.

Assessing risk should therefore involve all professions and involve a range of assessment criteria. It can be divided as risk to self and risk to others.

Risk to self through injurious behaviour invariably involves: past self-harm attempts (nature, motivations, dangerousness); presence and severity of current depression; presence of current suicidal ideation (method, ability to complete method, motivation); past and current drug or alcohol use; and past and current psychotic symptoms and their nature. In addition, an awareness of the strengths and limitations of the in-patient environment is crucial.

Risk to others includes assessment of the following: a known history of violence; the severity of previous violence; who the victims of violence were; thoughts of violence; previous and current psychotic symptoms and their nature (e.g., paranoia, command hallucinations); and past and current drug or alcohol use. Risk, however, should not be limited to physical violence as other risks may occur (e.g., threats, stalking, dangerous driving, etc.).

Assessing previous interventions

The responses to previous interventions are important but often overlooked. Knowledge of previous responses can determine whether the services have been appropriate for the patient and where weaknesses may lie. Consequently, the assessor should try to learn why the patient has returned to hospital from a global perspective and not merely from a diagnostic or symptom perspective. As such, the following is helpful:

- chronological history of previous interventions;
- the nature of these interventions;
- the means by which these interventions were delivered (length of admission, dose of medication, practitioner delivering);
- the known effectiveness of interventions (short-term and long-term effects and how these were measured);
- the patient's views of these interventions (acceptability, intrusiveness, satisfaction);
- previous and current medication (side-effects, adherence, cost).

How to assess

There are three methods of assessment – *interviewing, observation* and *measurement*. To increase the validity of assessments, assessors should incorporate all three, as reliance on only a single method introduces potential for bias. For example, observation provides an account of behaviours. It does not, however, account for motivations as these can only be determined through interviews. So, a comprehensive assessment collects complementary information, from which a broad insight into the patient's problems can be obtained.

Interviewing

The interview occupies a central place in the assessment process as it provides an opportunity for both the patient and the assessor to begin a therapeutic relationship. The initial face-to-face contact also enables the assessor to provide an orientation to the ward environment, guidance, information, engagement and reassurance that may be necessary according to the patient's needs (DoH, 2002). The interview enables the patient to state their problems in their own terms, thereby ensuring that their own views and experience are given central importance.

The assessment interview consists of a range of questions designed to help identify features of the patient's current experiences that are problematic or distressing. Of early importance is the patient's ability and willingness to be interviewed. Where patients are experiencing severe psychological distress, or are in need of physical interventions or observation, it is usually inappropriate to attempt to conduct a full interview. In these cases the nurse can utilise information from a number of other sources including carers, relatives and referrers, so that a detailed description of the patient's current functioning can be validated with the patient once their symptoms are controlled.

Assuming an interview can be carried out, it is essential that the assessor has the skills necessary to develop a therapeutic alliance and to be able to help the patient to manage any distress associated with both their symptoms and of being in an unfamiliar environment. Admission to a psychiatric unit alone may be a source of anxiety for patients and their families or carers. Thus, the assessor needs to show awareness of these emotions and to respond empathetically. Statements such as '*It seems as though you are finding this quite difficult at this time*' may be sufficient to indicate that the patient's distress has been acknowledged. Subsequent responses will vary according to the nature of distress the patient is experiencing, but is likely to include providing information and reassurance on the nature of the ward environment.

Applying Hawkins's (1986) 'funnelling' to the interview process the initial assessment involves the use of broad, open-ended questions such as

'*Can you tell me something about your recent experiences?*' or '*What was happening that resulted in your admission to hospital?*'

Once broad areas of functioning and experience have been identified, the assessor then selects those that are relevant to the patient's present admission. To facilitate this process it is useful to summarise the information that has been obtained, highlighting those that need to be explored in greater detail. This is helped by using the skills of paraphrasing, summarising and reflection. A typical question might include '*We've now got a lot of information on what has been happening for you, which is very helpful. You've said that you've been experiencing some difficult emotions lately – can you tell me some more about these?*'

As the interview progresses into the selective assessment stage, the style of questioning changes to more leading questions as these give the patient an indication of the nature of the information that is needed (Hawkins, 1986). For example, if open-ended questions result in responses that are too lengthy or discursive, a question such as '*You mentioned earlier that you've been feeling under pressure – can you tell me some more about this?*' may help to focus the response. Note that this question selects one of the patient's earlier responses and provides a prompt as to the areas of their experience about which information is sought. It is at this stage that more specific nursing models or diagnostic schemes may be utilised to provide some structure to information gathering, although it is still important to ensure that all psychological, social and biological areas of functioning are given consideration. Where indicated, semi-structured interviews are used to help identify relevant problems. If areas of functioning that are not directly related to the nurse's expertise are identified as warranting further attention, an initial management plan suggesting referral to other members of the ward team or other agencies should be developed.

The third stage of the interview process then focuses on the specific details of the problems identified (Hawkins, 1986). This is characterised by greater structure and may involve the use of closed questions to refine the interview process. Barker (1997) developed Kipling's Six Honest Serving Men, quoted at the beginning of this chapter, and suggests basing questions around the words, what, where, when, who, why, how, to obtain specific information regarding the patient's problems.

Observation

Observation is defined as

regarding the patient attentively while minimising the extent to which they feel under surveillance. (SNMAC, 1999: 2)

It is a key part of assessment and allows the assessor to test out hypotheses (e.g., does the patient appear to respond to hallucinations).

The Standing Nursing and Midwifery Advisory Committee (1999) classified observation into four levels.

- Level I: General observation.
- Level II: Intermittent observation.
- Level III: Within eyesight.
- Level IV: Within arm's length.

These are related to a procedure which is designed to manage risk, however, not to understand the patient. Observation, then, may be seen as both an assessment strategy and a management strategy, and it is important not to confuse the two. For the purpose of this chapter, observation is described as it relates to assessment.

Observing what patients say and do might appear to be one of the most straightforward approaches to assessment. In order to be done effectively and to produce meaningful accounts of patient's functioning, however, care needs to be taken in both the process of observing and reporting what was observed.

Observing behavioural symptoms

In observing behavioural symptoms, the purpose is to obtain precise descriptions of the behaviour with the minimum of inference or interpretation. Thus, when recording observations of behaviours, the actual behaviour should be described without attempting to ascribe a meaning. For example, just because a patient appears to be responding to auditory hallucinations does not mean that he or she is. As auditory hallucinations are only known to the patient, the only way to determine whether the behaviour is or is not a response to this is to ask the patient. In other words, here is a situation when methods of assessment must be mixed in order to understand why a patient behaves in a certain way.

Observing thoughts

It is not possible to observe patients' thoughts directly. (The same is true for other phenomena experienced by patients such as hallucinations, delusions, memories, flashbacks and other private events.) For this reason successful observation relies on the patient's verbal reports, or responses on specific questionnaires, to establish the existence of these symptoms. Of course, some emotional responses may be taken to indicate the presence of certain types of thoughts (e.g., crying may suggest the presence of negative thoughts, anxiety may suggest thoughts related to threat or danger), but the external observer cannot know what these thoughts are directly without asking the patient.

Asking the patient to identify and record various aspects of their thoughts/ experience is often a useful strategy. The process of *self-monitoring* engages the patient in their own care and has the additional advantage of being able to be done anywhere at any time, by the person who is experiencing the problem. Some care must, of course, be taken to ensure that the patient is able to engage in the process and that the effect is likely to be beneficial as, in some circumstances, asking a patient to focus on a symptom or thought might be associated with an increased amount of distress (e.g., command hallucinations, for which other assessment procedures might be better indicated). Effective self-monitoring requires an agreement with the patient of the precise behaviour or symptom to be recorded, along with methods for noting their occurrence. Common examples include thought diaries, ratings of mood throughout the day and activity diaries. One advantage of using self-monitoring as an assessment strategy is that the target symptom may sometimes decrease in frequency as a result. The main disadvantage of self-monitoring, however, is that it may lead to the patients producing the information that they feel the practitioner expects rather than being a reliable report of what actually occurred.

Observing physical symptoms

Observation of physical symptoms is generally reserved for those features of a patient's presentation that are related to some actual, objective physical reality such as blood pressure, motor activity or sleep. Other constructs that have a physiological component, but that are inferred through other behaviours (i.e., pain in the form of reaction to stimuli, hunger in the form of eating large amounts or stomach rumbling) may be better thought of as behaviours and assessed in that way (i.e., pain behaviour, hungry behaviour).

Observing social functioning

Direct observation of social functioning may be difficult within the acute in-patient environment, as the setting is obviously different from the patient's home. However, it may be appropriate to observe the patient's ability to engage in and perform activities of living. In practice, early assessment of these areas may be part of initial interviews, or be aided by rating scales, with more comprehensive assessment being conducted during later stages of the patient's stay in hospital.

Reporting the results of observation

Observations must be recorded accurately in order that the patient and multidisciplinary team can formulate and clarify the information obtained (Nursing and Midwifery Council, 2002). Consequently, observations should report what actually occurred in the situation. A useful rule-of-thumb is to ask whether another person would be able to accurately reproduce the behaviour described, given the description. This ensures that what is recorded retains some degree of objectivity and allows all members of the ward team reading the report to know what occurred even though they were not physically present. Although the use of diagnostic labels (e.g., schizophrenia, depression) and broad symptom labels (e.g., 'hallucinating') have use in professional communication, in reporting on observations they are of limited value. Therefore, for a patient who appeared to be responding to auditory hallucinations, a statement such as '*The patient was observed to be hallucinating*' would be better described as. '*The patient was observed looking at light switches and swearing at them on seven occasions this morning, following which he tried to disassemble one saying "They are in here"*'. Although this might seem laborious, the advantages of such detail are that it is individualised for the patient, and all who read the report will know precisely what occurred.

Limitations

Several factors should be considered when conducting, reporting and understanding the results of observation. The first relates to whether all those involved in the observation interpret and record the behaviour in the same way. This is known as *inter-observer agreement* and it is important in acute in-patient environments where more than one member of the ward team conducts observational procedures. One way to ensure that inter-observer agreement is high is to ensure that the behaviours or symptoms of interest are clearly specified in the patient's care plan and that the methods for recording are understood and accessible to all observers.

The second factor relates to whether the same observer will reliably produce similar accounts of the same behaviour conducted at different times or in different settings *intra-observer agreement*. Ensuring that the assessor is able to carry out the procedure without distractions and with a clear understanding of what is being assessed can enhance this.

The frequencies that the behaviour is recorded must also be considered. Observing and recording events that occur at a high rate, such as checking rituals in Obsessive Compulsive Disorder (OCD), may result in copious amounts of repeated information. To overcome this it is often useful to record the behaviours that occur within a given time frame. Similarly, attempting to observe behaviours that are relatively low in frequency may use up a large amount of observer time for only one or two occurrences. In such circumstances it is useful to use role-play methods where the patient is asked to perform the behaviour, even though it is not a natural occurrence.

Finally, the effect of the observer on the patient and their behaviour must be recognised. In some cases the behaviour or symptoms that are being assessed will alter simply because of the presence of the observer. This is known as *reactivity*. Again, some patients with OCD report little or no urge to conduct rituals when they are being observed. This is because they rationalise that the observer will take responsibility should a catastrophe result from the ritual not being performed. On the other hand, other patients may appear more agitated, anxious and aggressive if they are aware that their behaviour is being regularly monitored.

Measurement

Conducted on admission, measurement procedures provide a baseline from which future changes may be compared. It may also assist other assessment procedures to identify relevant problem areas. Some measurements are based on a patient's score on a specific questionnaire or rating scale and are used to help arrive at a diagnosis.

As with interviewing and observation, measurement may be made at a number of levels. The most general comprises broad assessment questionnaires which are used to assess psychological, physical or social functioning.

- Global Assessment of Functioning (GAF) (American Psychiatric Association, 1994). A clinician-rated 0–100 scale that assesses symptom severity or level of psychological, social and occupational functioning where non-organic psychological symptoms are present.
- Health of the Nation Outcome Scales (HoNOS) (Wing et al., 1998). This 12-item scale, intended for use by nurses and psychiatrists, examines both clinical problems and social functioning. It is discussed fully in Chapter 2 of this book.

Domain-specific measures identify the presence of symptoms, or level of functioning, within the parameters of the selected domain. Domains are defined by concepts such as level of social functioning, or the parameters of the patient's medical diagnosis (e.g., depression, schizophrenia). These are sometimes referred to as nomothetic assessment procedures, as they are intended to apply to all patients within the selected group.

Measures for the domain of medical diagnoses

- **Schizophrenia**

  o Positive and Negative Syndrome Scale for Schizophrenia (PANNS) (Kay et al., 1992). Assesses psychotic and related symptoms and gives three sub-scale scores for positive, negative and general symptoms.
  o Signs and Symptoms of Psychotic Illness (SSPI) (Liddle et al., 2002). A 20-item clinician-rated scale. Nineteen of the items assess the presence of symptoms in five areas commonly seen in psychotic illness. These are depression, excitation, diminished psychomotor activity and reality distortion; one item assesses insight.

- **Obsessive Compulsive Disorder (OCD)**

  o Yale–Brown Obsessive Compulsive Scale (YBOCS) (Goodman et al., 1989a, 1989b). A 10-item clinician-administered semi-structured interview and 64-item clinician-administered checklist designed to measure the severity and types of symptoms in Obsessive Compulsive Disorder. Ratings result in an overall score and ratings of severity for obsessions and compulsions. A self-report version has also been developed (Baer, 2000).
  o Maudsley Obsessional Compulsive Inventory (MOCI) (Hodgson and Rachman, 1977). A 30-item self-report scale, with items being rated as 'True' or 'False'. Scores on four sub-scales can be obtained (cleaning, slowness, doubting, checking) in addition to an overall score.

- **Bipolar Disorder**

  o Young Mania Rating Scale (YMRS) (Young et al., 1978). An 11-item, clinician-administered rating scale that assesses the various symptoms of mania on a 0 to 4 scale, where 0 = absent and 4 = the most severe.

- **Depression**

  o Beck Depression Inventory (BDI) (Beck et al., 1961; Beck and Steer, 1987). The original questionnaire is a 21-item rating scale completed by patients. Items cover the main symptoms of depression in the form of statements and respondents are asked to mark the presence of each symptom over the last week. Items are scored on a 0 to 4 scale.
  o Zung Self-Rating Depression Scale (ZSDS) (Zung and Durham, 1965). The Beck Depression Inventory and the ZSDS are the main self-administered instruments for the assessment of depression.

These scales are often used as 'screening tools' and not as substitutes for an in-depth interview.

- **Post-traumatic Stress Disorder**

  o Impact of Events Scale (IES) (Horowitz et al., 1979; Sundin and Horowitz, 2002). A 15-item self-report scale that assesses symptoms of intrusion and avoidance following a traumatic event.

  o Clinician-Administered PTSD Scale (CAPS) (Blake et al., 1995). The items relate to the DSM-IV (APA, 1994) criteria for PTSD; i.e., re-experiencing, avoidance and increased arousal, duration of over a month and interference with functioning.

Measures for the domain of social functioning

- The Camberwell Assessment of Need (CAN) (Slade et al., 1999). Assesses the health and social needs of people with mental health problems. The clinical version of the scale for adults assesses needs and help across 22 areas. Level of need is identified along with the level of help required and already received, and satisfaction with the help received.
- The Work and Social Adjustment Scale (WASS) (Marks, 1986; Mundt et al., 2002). A five-item self-report scale that assesses 'functional impairment attributable to an identified problem' (p. 461) in the areas of work, home management, social leisure activities, private leisure activities, and ability to form and maintain close relationships with others. Responses for each item are rated on a 0 to 8 scale, where 0 = not at all impaired and 8 = very severely impaired.

Measures for the domain of quality of life

- The World Health Organisation Quality of Life Assessment 100-item version (WHO-QOL-100) (WHOQOL Group, 1998). A generic measure that assesses quality of life across six domains; specifically: physical, psychological, independence, social relationships, environment and spirituality. Each domain has a number of 'facets' resulting in a 100-item scale.
- Schizophrenia Quality of Life Scale (SQLS) (Wilkinson et al., 2000). A 30-item self-report instrument that comprises three scales: psychosocial, motivation, and energy, symptoms and side-effects.

Measures for the domain of risk assessment

- The HCR-20 (Webster et al., 1995) was developed as a 'broadband' violence risk assessment tool. The conceptual scheme of the HCR-20 identifies 'markers' for previous, current and future risk. 'HCR' is an acronym for Historical, Clinical and Risk management variables. The Historical variables represent the more or less static ground factors included in earlier actuarial tools. The Clinical variables are meant to reflect risk in light of current presentation, state of symptoms, insight and attitudes. The Risk management variables represent a systematised appraisal of future risk, including plan feasibility, social network support and contextual factors. For a comprehensive review see Webster et al. (1997), Douglas et al. (1999) and Dolan and Doyle (2000).

Finally, individualised measures are used that are based on the individual patient and their problems. These are known as idiographic assessments as they use the patient's own data to provide information on what to assess.

- **Measuring behaviour.** Accurate measurement of behaviour is closely related to observation. Observation procedures produce a clear specification of the behaviour to be measured so that instances of its occurrence can be identified. Once this has been done, the most common aspects of a patient's behaviour to measure are the frequency, the duration, the *intensity* and the *latency* (Martin and Bateson, 1993).

  - *Frequency* refers to the number of times something happens in a given time; for example, the number of checks per day or the number of times someone has attempted to leave the ward in one shift.
  - *Duration* indicates how long each episode of behaviour lasts; for example, the amount of time spent outside of the room.
  - *Intensity* of behaviour is sometimes difficult to define and measure (Martin and Bateson, 1993) but may be used to describe variations in similar behaviours; for example, angry behaviour showing differing intensities through variation in the number of expletives used.
  - *Latency* refers to the amount of time from a specific event to the onset of behaviour. This may be of particular interest in problems where people report an inability to resist urges, such as OCD or impulse control disorders, where increasing the time between urge and act may be an initial focus of treatment. A common use of latency is in the area of sleep disorders where the amount of time between going to bed and falling asleep (*sleep-onset latency*) is often used to assess the effectiveness of treatments.

- **Measuring thoughts.** Measuring the occurrence of thoughts is difficult as they are not physically observable and therefore need to be reported by the patient. Some methods are available to assess the frequency of thoughts. The most straightforward is the thought diary. Thought diaries require the patient to note down the content of specific thoughts as and when they occur. The assessment focuses on the person's *automatic thoughts* that reflect their ongoing appraisals of events in their lives. Alternatively, if the frequency of specific thoughts is of interest, the patient may be given a 'clicker-counter' in order to provide a numerical estimate.

Limitations

Conducting measurements using questionnaires, checklists and rating scales is a useful part of the assessment process. However, it is important that the questionnaires that are used measure what they are supposed to. The scales referenced in this chapter are supported by research-based evidence detailing their development and use. These are their psychometric properties and particularly focus on two areas: validity and reliability.

The validity of a questionnaire or rating scale refers to whether or not it assesses what it is intended to. Two main aspects should be considered: face validity and content validity (Streiner and Norman, 1995). Face validity is the clinician's initial judgement as to whether the scale assesses the problem or disorder adequately. Content validity adds to face validity by assessing whether the scale consists of enough items to cover the problem or disorder. For example, a five-item scale for depression might have some face validity if it asks questions on mood, energy, motivation, concentration and appetite, because these features do occur in depression. Its content validity would be increased if it also assessed suicidal ideation, sleep patterns and activity levels as these also occur in depressed patients. Therefore, when using a scale it is often helpful to ask, 'Does this scale look like it covers the problem area or disorder?' and 'Does this scale cover enough of the symptoms to make it useful to the assessment of this patient?'

Reliability refers to whether a questionnaire produces similar results, when used on the same people on different occasions, or by different observers. This is important as practitioners need to be sure that the measurement procedure itself does not influence the scores produced by the scales.

Unfortunately there are many questionnaires available that have not been developed scientifically. The danger is that they may not return the results they are supposed to or, more dangerously, they may return inaccurate results.

Sources of information

Assessment information can be obtained from a variety of sources (patient, carer/family, referrer) and in a number of ways (letters, verbal reports,

Table 1.1 Methods of assessment and sources of information

		Primary	Secondary
Method	Direct	Observation of current behaviour/symptoms by patient or trained observer	Observation of behaviour/symptoms by others
	Indirect	Interview with patient. Patient questionnaires and other measurement procedures	Case-notes, reports referral letters

case-notes). Each source is useful, according to the type of information being sought, and they are categorised into primary or secondary sources. Primary sources of information are patients, as they are the ones who experience the problem and are best placed to report on what is happening to them first-hand. Secondary sources of information are the assessor, families, and carers and referrers. These provide information on behaviour or symptoms that have already occurred.

It is also necessary to make a distinction between direct and indirect methods of assessment (see Table 1.1). Direct methods report what actually occurred as and when it happened. Well-conducted observations are the best form of direct assessment as they limit the amount of time between the occurrence of the symptom and its recording. Indirect methods, on the other hand, are those that give accounts of behaviour, symptoms or problems that occurred at some other time or place. Interviews are indirect because they usually give accounts of what *has* happened and therefore rely on the information being historically accurate. Questionnaires and rating scales are also indirect methods as they convert information from the patient into numerical scores and/or agreement with pre-written statements. Similarly, all secondary sources of information are indirect as they also report on what happened previously. Consequently, when reporting the results of assessment, it is always useful to state the source of the information, as well the method used to obtain it, so that the information can be placed in its appropriate context.

Planning

To emphasise the involvement of service users within contemporary mental health care, as well as being recorded in the patients' records, written copies of care plans should also be provided to patients and their families or carers (DoH, 2000, 2002).

Using the information derived from the assessment, care planning focuses on two areas. The first is to develop strategies that are designed to manage the patient's care, and the second develops plans designed to provide therapeutic interventions.

Management plans are predominantly devised to take into account the overall procedures and systems of care that provide the framework for the patient's stay in hospital. A comprehensive management care plan specifies:

- who the patient's named nurse is;
- level of observation required;
- the Care Programme Approach level including review dates and the names of all those involved in the patient's care;
- whether any restrictions apply to the patient according to their status under the Mental Health Act 1983;
- other agencies that are to be involved or to whom the patient has been referred;
- the family's or carer's perspective, involvement and information needs;
- known risk factors and how they should be predicted, managed and communicated.

The second type of plan is a treatment or intervention care plan. This is designed to address the specific bio-psycho-social problems identified at assessment with the interventions that are to be implemented. A comprehensive treatment care plan is provided for each identified problem and includes:

- a clear statement of the problem including relevant results from measurement procedures;
- the treatment goals;
- the treatment interventions that are to be used;
- who is responsible for conducting the treatment;
- methods for monitoring the patient's progress;
- the family's or carer's involvement in the treatment.

It is crucial that the differences between management and intervention plans are understood. Management plans do not necessarily intervene or assist to change a person's problems. They are solely a management strategy whereas intervention plans only consider therapeutic interventions. An abundance of one type of care plan in the absence of another may indicate the need to re-examine the patient's assessment to ensure that all areas of need have been identified and that all facets of care are considered.

Conclusion

This chapter has provided an overview of the assessment process in acute in-patient settings. The chapter has examined the broad principles and practice of assessment using the three methods of interviewing, observing and measurement.

In discussing assessment, applications within the acute psychiatric in-patient environment have been provided. However, it is impossible to examine all the factors that are at play when assessing. For example, local environmental factors such as the behaviour of other patients on the ward or staff shortages, will influence the assessment findings. In addition, despite attempts to standardise assessment tools, because of the interpretive element of assessment, the experience and knowledge of the assessor will also influence the outcome. Nonetheless, the issues remain the same; that is, that the assessment is the aspect which determines future care, management and intervention. For this reason it is crucial that the assessment is as accurate as possible. The better the assessment the more likely the chance of a successful outcome for the patient.

References

American Psychiatric Association (1994) *Diagnostic and Statistical Manual of Mental Disorders*, 4th edn. Washington, DC: American Psychiatric Association.

Baer, L. (2000) *Getting Control: Overcoming your Obsessions and Compulsion.* New York: Plume.

Barker, P.J. (1997) *Assessment in Psychiatric and Mental Health Nursing: In Search of the Whole Person.* Cheltenham: Nelson Thornes.

Barker, P.J. (2002) 'The Tidal Model: the healing potential of metaphor within the patient's narrative', *Journal of Psychosocial Nursing*, 40 (7): 42–50.

Beck, A.T. and Steer, R.A. (1987) *Manual for the Revised Beck Depression Inventory.* San Antonio: Psychological Corporation.

Beck, A.T., Ward, C.H., Mendelson, M., Mock, J.E. and Erbaugh, J.K. (1961) 'An inventory for measuring depression', *Archives of General Psychiatry*, 4: 561–71.

Blake, D.D., Weathers, F.W., Nagy, L.M., Kaloupek, D.G., Gusman, F.D., Charney, D.S., and Keane, T.M. (1995) 'The development of a clinician administered PTSD scale', *Journal of Traumatic Stress*, 8: 75–90.

Douglas, K., Cox, D. and Webster, C. (1999) 'Violence risk assessment: science and practice', *Legal and Criminological Psychology*, 4: 184–94.

Department of Health (1999) *National Service Framework for Mental Health – Delivering Modern Standards for Mental Health.* London: The Stationery Office.

Department of Health (2000) *Effective Care Co-ordination in Mental Health Services: Modernising the Care Programme Approach – A Policy Booklet.* London: The Stationery Office.

Department of Health (2002) *Mental Health Policy Implementation Guide: Adult Acute In-patient Care Provision.* London: The Stationery Office.

Dolan, M. and Doyle, M. (2000) 'Violence risk prediction: clinical and actuarial measures and the role of the psychopathy checklist', *British Journal of Psychiatry*, 177: 303–11.

Goodman, W.K., Price, L.H., Rasmussen, S.A., Mazure, C., Fleischmann, R.L., Hill, C.L., Heninger, G.R. and Charney, D.S. (1989a) 'The Yale–Brown Obsessive Compulsive Scale: I. Development, use and reliability', *Archives of General Psychiatry*, 46: 1006–11.

Goodman, W.K., Price, L.H., Rasmussen, S.A., Mazure, C., Delgado, P., Heninger, G.R., and Charney, D.S. (1989b) 'The Yale–Brown Obsessive Compulsive Scale: II. Validity', *Archives of General Psychiatry*, 46: 1012–16.

Hawkins, R.P. (1986) 'Selection of target behaviours', in R.O. Nelson, and S.C. Hayes, (eds), *Conceptual Foundations of Behavioral Assessment*. New York: Guilford Press.

Hodgson, R.J. and Rachman, S. (1977) 'Obsessive compulsive complaints', *Behaviour Research and Therapy*, 15: 389–95.

Horowitz, M., Wilner, N. and Alvarez, W. (1979) 'Impact of event scale: a measure of subjective distress', *Psychosomatic Medicine*, 41: 209–18.

Kay, S.R., Opler, L.A., and Fiszbein, A. (1992) *Positive and Negative Syndrome Scale*. New York: Multi-Health Systems.

Liddle, P.F., Ngan, E.T.C., Duffield, G., Kho, K. and Warren, A.J. (2002) 'Signs and symptoms of psychotic illness scale (SSPI): a rating scale', *British Journal of Psychiatry*, 180: 45–50.

Marks, I.M. (1986) *Behavioural Psychotherapy*. Bristol: John Wright.

Martin, P. and Bateson, P. (1993) *Measuring Behaviour: An Introductory Guide*. Cambridge: Cambridge University Press.

Maslow, A. (1954) *Motivation and Personality*. New York: Harper.

Mathes, E. (1981) 'Maslow's hierarchy of needs as a guide for living', *Journal of Humanistic Psychology*, 21: 69–72.

Mundt, J.C., Marks, I.M., Shear, K., and Greist, J.H. (2002) 'The Work and Social Adjustment Scale: a simple measure of impairment in functioning', *British Journal of Psychiatry*, 180: 461–4.

Nursing and Midwifery Council (2002) *Guidelines for Record Keeping*. London: Nursing and Midwifery Council.

Sainsbury Centre for Mental Health (SCMH) (2001) *The Capable Practitioner*. London: Sainsbury Centre for Mental Health.

Slade, M., Loftus, L., Phelan, M., Thornicroft, G. and Wykes, T. (1999) *The Camberwell Assessment of Need*. London: Gaskell.

Standing Nursing and Midwifery Advisory Committee (SNMAC) (1999) *Practice Guidance: Safe and Supportive Observation of Patients at Risk*. London: The Stationery Office.

Streiner, D.L. and Norman, G.R. (1995) *Health Measurement Scales: A Practical Guide to their Development and Use*. Oxford: Oxford Medical Publications.

Sundin, E.C. and Horowitz, M.J. (2002) 'Impact of Event Scale: psychometric properties', *British Journal of Psychiatry*, 180: 205–9.

Webster, C., Harris, G., Rice, M., Cormier, C. and Quinsey, V. (1995) *The HCR-20 Scheme: The Assessment of Dangerousness and Risk*. Vancouver: Simon Fraser University and British Columbia Forensic Psychiatric Services Commission.

Webster, C.D., Douglas, K.S., Eaves, D. and Hart, S.D. (1997) 'Assessing risk of violence to others', in *Impulsivity: Theory Assessment and Treatment*. New York: Guilford Press.

WHOQOL Group (1998) 'The World Health Organisation Quality of Life Assessment (WHOQOL): development and psychometric properties', *Social Science and Medicine*, 46: 1569–85.

Wilkinson, G., Hesdon, B., Wild, D., Cookson, R., Farina, C., Sharma, V., Fitzpatrick, R. and Jenkinson, C. (2000) 'Self-report quality of life measure for people with schizophrenia: the SQLS', *British Journal of Psychiatry*, 177: 42–6.

Wing, J.K., Beevor, A.S., Curtis, R.H., Park, S.B.G., Hadden, S. and Burns, A. (1998) 'Health of the Nation Outcome Scales (HoNOS): research and development', *British Journal of Psychiatry*, 172: 11–18.

Workforce Action Team (2001) *Mental Health National Service Framework and NHS Plan. Workforce Planning, Education and Training Underpinning Project: Adult Mental Health Services. Final Report.* London: Department of Health.

Young, R.C., Biggs, J.T., Ziegler, V.E., and Meyer, D.A. (1978) 'A rating scale for mania: reliability, validity and sensitivity', *British Journal of Psychiatry*, 133: 429–35.

Zung W.W. and Durham, N.C. (1965) 'A self-rating depression scale', *Archives of General Psychiatry*, 12: 63–70.

TWO

Measuring health and social functioning using HoNOS

Mick James and Damian Mitchell

Introduction

Measuring the outcomes of mental health care can potentially be achieved using a wide variety of measures. Thornicroft and Tansella (1996) provide a broad overview of potential measures that includes measures of quality of life, carer burden, patient satisfaction and assessment of need. It can be argued that not all of these represent a measurement of outcome in the purest sense, but it is important to remember that a large range of measures exist which may be potentially useful in measuring the outcome of acute in-patient care. It can also be argued that it would be impractical to use a number of these measures in a routine clinical setting such as an acute in-patient unit, since the task would be very time-consuming. This aside, some of these measures may be worthy of consideration for use in periodic surveys or more specific enquiries within an in-patient unit.

A report by a working group to the Department of Health (Charlwood et al., 1999) provides a series of recommendations on outcome indicators for severe mental illness. These have since been incorporated as part of the National Service Framework for Mental Health Services (Department of Health, 1999). A number of the recommended outcome indicators make use of Health of the Nation Outcome Scales (HoNOS) (Wing et al., 1996) and it is the use of these scales within an acute in-patient unit that is the focus of this chapter. They are simple and easy to use in routine clinical practice and represent a feasible starting point for the measurement of outcome in mental health services to be tackled.

Background to the development of the scales

As its name suggests the HoNOS project sprang from the government White Paper *The Health of the Nation* (Department of Health, 1992), which included mental ill-health as one of the five key areas in its strategy for promoting the health of the population. *The Health of the Nation* document identified three targets that specifically related to mental health, namely:

To improve significantly the health and social functioning of mentally ill people

To reduce the overall suicide rate by at least 15% by the year 2000 (from 11.0 per 100,000 population in 1990 to no more than 9.4)

To reduce the suicide rate of severely mentally ill people by at least 33% by the year 2000 (from the life-time estimate of 15% in 1990 to no more than 10%)

(Department of Health, 1993: 11)

The latter two targets can be seen to be more measurable than the first in that they deal with quantitative data that are collected and collated nationally and therefore in principle easier to make calculations of progress or lack of it (however, in practice, difficulties did arise due to the nature of how data on unnatural deaths were recorded). The first mental health target, by comparison, offers little in the way of clear-cut variables as the terminology used is ill-defined. For example, what is meant by the term 'health' or 'mental illness' and which 'mentally ill people' are we concerned with? The rather nebulous nature of this target led, in 1993, to the Department of Health commissioning the Royal College of Psychiatrists' Research Unit (CRU) to come up with a set of scales that would allow measurement of progress against this first mental health target.

The CRU began by establishing a multidisciplinary working group to advise on the project. This was an important consideration as it was always intended from the outset to be a measure that could and should be used by all qualified mental health professionals. The initial phase of the project determined that no existing measure could adequately do the job. Whilst there were numerous measures of health and measures of social functioning, no one single measure offered a sufficiently broad coverage of both which was suitable for use in routine clinical practice. A number of existing scales were designed predominantly as research instruments and were therefore too lengthy and time-consuming for use in routine clinical practice. It became clear that a new measure would have to be developed that incorporated a number of key elements. Namely that it would have to be viewed by mental health professionals as relevant and practical in terms of their own needs to record and monitor client data and that it could not be a time-consuming or complex instrument. This latter point was seen as particularly

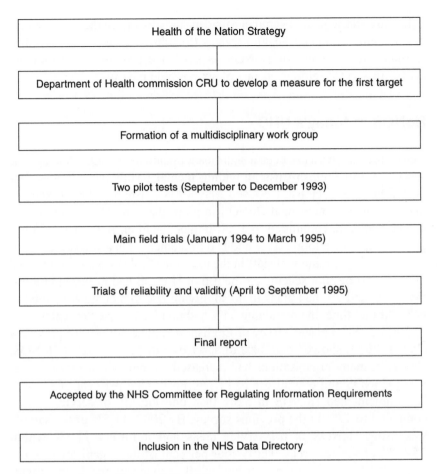

Figure 2.1   Development of HoNOS

significant, as it was recognised that busy clinicians would not accept and would be unlikely to implement a long and cumbersome instrument in their day-to-day practice. Despite the need for brevity, it was also acknowledged that any such instrument would have to be shown to be sensitive to change over time, stand up in terms of reliability and validity and therefore be sufficiently robust to provide sound aggregated data that could inform public health planning (Wing et al., 1996). HoNOS was subsequently constructed and underwent extensive testing and refining in field trials over a period of three years. The upshot was a final version (HoNOS 4) that was considered and accepted by the Committee for Regulating Information Requirements and entered into the NHS Data Dictionary in 1996 (see Figure 2.1).

In Australia, a large government-funded study to look at the measurement of outcomes in mental health services (Steadman et al., 1997) has also recommended the use of HoNOS as a service provider-rated measure across all service settings, as one of six possible measures.

HoNOS in today's NHS

Across the UK there has been a significant uptake of HoNOS. A telephone survey of 140 English trusts providing mental health services was conducted between October 1997 and May 1998 (Bishop, 1998). It showed that 17% had implemented HoNOS in more than one locality or service setting and were committed to a full implementation. A further 16% had gone beyond the piloting stage and had implemented in a single locality or service setting. Training of staff in the use of the scales who were involved in some sort of pilot scheme on the use of HoNOS had occurred in a further 26%, and 7% had plans to do so, giving rise to a cumulative total of 66%. At that time, the remaining 34% had no plans to use the scales.

A more recent postal survey of English mental health service providers (James, 2002) showed that 34% of services still had no use of HoNOS. However, many organisations had increased the number of service areas using HoNOS and overall use had risen. Forty-nine per cent of services had implemented HoNOS in more than one locality or service setting compared to 17% in the previous survey. By 2002, 11.5% of the sample was using HoNOS in *all* service areas and a further 11.5% within 75–99% of service areas. Thirty-four per cent of the organisations were using HoNOS routinely in over half of all service settings. In the organisations where routine use was identified, 79% of nurses were using HoNOS. Within other staff groups 59% of occupational therapists, 53% of social workers, 26.5% of psychologists and 23.5% of medical staff were using HoNOS routinely. Within services with routine use of HoNOS, 68% were undertaking ratings at CPA reviews, and ratings were undertaken at ward admission and ward discharge in 59% of these services (James, 2002).

In addition, the CRU has sent out in excess of 10,000 scales and glossaries to around 90 services over the last few years and continues to coordinate training, providing training services to a further 25 trusts. In addition, HoNOS has now achieved an international profile, having been translated into a number of different languages (Wing et al., 2000).

It might perhaps have been anticipated that take-up of HoNOS would have been more widespread by 2002 but a number of factors may have militated against this. The most obvious being the change of government in the UK during the intervening period from commissioning to completion of the HoNOS project. However, commitment to outcome measurement did not wane at the Department of Health following the change in administration. On the contrary, attempts to ensure that outcome measurement became an integral part of Mental Health services in the UK continued apace and interest in HoNOS was re-kindled. For instance, the working group, commissioned by the Department of Health in 1996 to advise on indicators of health outcomes for individuals with severe mental illness (Charlwood et al., 1999), describe a number of the measures of outcome, several of which use HoNOS data. A summary of these is also contained in an annex to the National Service Framework for Mental Health which states that HoNOS will be incorporated into the Mental Health Minimum Data Set (MHMDS) (NHS Information Authority, 2000) as part of the mental health information strategy.

The working group defined severe mental illness as follows:

- there must be a mental disorder as designated by a mental health professional (psychiatrist, mental health nurse, clinical psychologist, occupational therapist or mental health social worker) and either
- there must have been a score of 4 (very severe problem) on at least one, or a score of 3 (moderately severe problem) on at least two, of the HoNOS items 1–10 (excluding item 5 'physical illness or disability problems') during the previous six months or
- there must have been a significant level of service usage over the past five years as shown by:

  1. a total of six months in a psychiatric ward or day hospital, or
  2. three admissions to hospital or day hospital, or
  3. six months of psychiatric community care involving more than one worker or the perceived need for such care if unavailable or refused.

(Department of Health, 1999: 126)

This means that, in effect, HoNOS scores will be a consideration in how 'severe mental illness' is defined. One of the outcome indicators is an annual assessment of the number of people meeting this definition divided by the size of the local population. The rationale for this measure is that it may be possible to prevent some mental health problems from worsening to the point where the individual becomes severely mentally ill, and this would provide a measure of success in trying to do this.

As a result of this association with the definition of SMI, HoNOS scores are implicit in a number of the outcome indicators recommended by Charlwood et al. (1999). One of these looks at admission to an in-patient unit on detection of SMI. The indicator states that for a local population in any given year, the number of people meeting the criteria of SMI referred to earlier, 'whose first contact with mental health services coincides with an in-patient psychiatric admission occurring within the given year, divided by the total number of people meeting the diagnostic and

HoNOS criteria for SMI presenting for the first time to mental health services, in the given year' (Charlwood et al., 1999: 23). The rationale for this is that, ideally, people developing SMI should be detected and treated promptly by community services, thus avoiding the need for an acute in-patient admission.

There are two outcome indicators in which the use of HoNOS data are more explicit and these may provide a useful starting point in using HoNOS data locally. The first of these looks at the HoNOS scores for the whole of a service providers' population of individuals with SMI. It provides guidance on the use of HoNOS data to assess the ability of a whole service to improve or maintain the functioning of individuals with SMI, with the aim of reducing the need for these individuals to receive acute in-patient care. The methodology described is likely to be valuable in making comparisons between service providers and in the analysis of trends over time within a local service population. It is recognised that it may be of limited use within an acute in-patient setting (Charlwood et al., 1999: 25–7). The second of these outcome indicators looks specifically at acute in-patient populations and is described in full in the section on the uses of HoNOS.

Collecting information on the use of mental health services is not new. Much of the information that is assembled in the MHMDS is currently already being collected from a variety of sources, including the Hospital Episode Statistics (HES), the Common Information Core (CIC) and the Korner aggregated returns. However, these are all in aggregated form rather than being related to individual service use episodes. The MHMDS will provide a standard record of a client's experience of services focusing on the clinical process. It will comprise a variety of data about the individual, including demographic information, details of the care provided and the way this care is managed, as well as diagnoses and the HoNOS ratings for that individual. Assessment of outcome is a cornerstone of this new dataset with HoNOS providing this key outcome data. As part of the MHMDS HoNOS ratings will be required for the following times:

- first in spell
- most recent in spell
- worst in spell
- best in reporting period

(Department of Health, 1997)

The Mental Health Information Strategy (MHIS) sets out a progressive agenda, with the intention that '[By] 2005 professionals in primary, secondary and social care, together with the public, service users and their carers will have timely, accurate and appropriate access to the mental health information they need' (Department of Health, 2001: 3). This document has, at its heart, the intention of improving how information is collated and used within Mental Health services and maps out the actions necessary to achieve the information requirements of the *National Service Framework for Mental Health* (Department of Health, 1999) and *Information for Health* (Secretary of State, 1998). HoNOS is identified as the key outcome indicator, which as part of an MHMDS can help to meet the goal of providing 'quality and management information to aid continuous service improvement' (Department of Health, 2001: 30). It is clear, therefore, that HoNOS will become a necessary part of data collection and performance management for mental health services in the UK for the foreseeable future. The challenge for mental health professionals is to ensure that it is used appropriately to provide useful, timely, quality data for managing client caseloads and targeting activities and resources to meet client needs.

What is HoNOS?

HoNOS is a short, simple set of scales that provides a profile and measure of the severity of an individual's behavioural, impairment and mental health problems as well as their current social functioning. The scales are designed for use in any setting in secondary mental health care services and are based on a rating of the worst symptoms/problems that have occurred during the previous two-week period. As HoNOS was principally designed as a health outcome measure, ratings have to be made on at least two occasions in order to determine whether an individual has improved, deteriorated or stayed the same over the intervening period. When more than two ratings are made it then provides a means of examining trends over time, both for individuals and groups of individuals.

The scales cover a broad range of elements that constitute health and social functioning and are intended to be completed in a few minutes by clinicians after routine clinical assessments (most usually at CPA reviews or ward rounds). The rating thus obtained provides a brief numerical record of the clinical assessment in terms of the current health and social functioning of the individual. Once two ratings have been made for an individual, the differences between the levels of severity provide a measure of outcome, but it is important to note that this is a measure of mental health outcome for that individual, not the health care outcomes as a result of the care and treatment provided.

HoNOS provides a standard record of progress across 12 common types of problem. Once the scores have been recorded they provide a quick checklist for clinicians to refer to in their routine clinical practice. Experience has shown that it is easy to incorporate into existing services and structures, as an integral part of CPA reviews, and as part of the admission and discharge process in acute in-patient areas (James and Kehoe, 1999). It can be used as a means of comparing health outcomes against those expected as a result of clinical intervention. It can also provide a standardised tool for audit or for clinical research. Finally, it can be used as a method of matching patient needs to the skills of practitioners, and as a means of examining casemix and caseload (Wing et al., 1996).

What HoNOS is not

Equally important is to consider what HoNOS is not, as inappropriate use of the tool has often led to confusion and rejection of the instrument by clinical staff. HoNOS is not a structured clinical assessment tool or interview guide, which means that staff should not take the client through each item in turn by asking questions relating to each. That said, a thorough assessment is a prerequisite to undertaking a HoNOS rating, as a sound knowledge of the client's level of functioning over the previous two-week period is essential. A HoNOS rating should be made immediately following the clinician's routine assessment, whether that is the initial interview, follow-up or pre-discharge. However, some staff may find that their usual method of assessment does not provide them with all the data required to make a rating and therefore some slight adjustments to the way in which assessments are conducted may be necessary.

Also, in recognition that HoNOS provides only one aspect of outcome data, it should be strongly asserted that HoNOS ratings should not be seen as a substitute or replacement for clinical notes. What staff discuss with and write about their clients will always be the most important source of evidence on which clinicians will base their judgements. Background material, in the shape of qualitative descriptions, is also necessary to put HoNOS ratings in perspective when considering an individual's progression (or lack of it).

HoNOS ratings do not provide an assessment of future risk as it was not designed as a risk assessment tool but clearly HoNOS has implications for risk management as a number of the items relate to known risk indicators. For example, if a client scores as having a severe or very severe problem in relation to item 1 on the scale, *Overactive, aggressive, disruptive or agitated behaviour*, then clearly staff have a professional responsibility to act on that data to protect the client and/or others. So information obtained from HoNOS ratings needs to be considered in risk assessment and risk management protocols. It is important to note that all acute in-patient clients should have an assessment of risk as part of the admission process.

HoNOS ratings do not measure health care outcomes or clinical effectiveness (e.g., interventions), due to the broad-spectrum nature of the instrument (i.e., changes in the client's circumstances may alter the ratings which have little to do with clinical interventions). There are a great number of ways to measure more specific health outcomes, such as psychotic symptoms or depressed mood, and HoNOS does not represent a substitute for any of these more specific, standardised assessment tools or rating scales. What HoNOS does provide is a measure of health and social functioning (health and social outcome) for an individual client or groups of clients, and of course HoNOS data can and should be used *alongside* other outcome data to make decisions about clinical effectiveness. Most particularly the scores from the sub-sets of the HoNOS rating may prove more clinically relevant than the overall score, as *'behavioural problems'*, *'impairment problems'* and *'symptomatic problems'* are obvious targets for clinical intervention. Aggregated data from the sub-sets, used alongside other more specific scales may prove a valuable addition to clinical outcome measurement.

Finally, HoNOS is not a decision-making tool or a substitute for an MDS (minimum dataset), though if used as part of an MDS it may prove useful for informing the decision-making process. Although HoNOS was not designed for this purpose and therefore offers only partial information, as with the measurement of clinical outcome, used alongside other data and placed in context HoNOS data can play a part in the planning of service provision or resource allocation though it should always be used with caution and with expert advice.

HoNOS structure and use

The scale consists of 12 items, which are rated consecutively, the order in which they are listed being intended to reflect the likely severity with which the problems impact on an individual's health and social functioning. Each item is rated using the same severity scale that has five points:

0 No problem
1 Minor problem requiring no action
2 Mild problem but definitely present
3 Moderately severe problem
4 Severe to very severe problem

NB: '9' is used to denote that not enough data are available to make a rating but has no numerical value (i.e. is not counted in the overall score).

A glossary provides information on each of the items and examples of current 'health' status for each of the points on the severity scale.

The 12 HoNOS items

1. Overactive, aggressive, disruptive or agitated behaviour.
2. Non-accidental self-injury.
3. Problem drinking or drug-taking.
4. Cognitive problems.
5. Physical illness or disability problems.
6. Problems associated with hallucinations and delusions.
7. Problems with depressed mood.
8. Other mental and behavioural problems.
9. Problems with relationships.
10. Problems with activities of daily living.
11. Problems with living conditions.
12. Problems with occupation and activities.

Since HoNOS contains 12 items which are each scored from 0 to 4 on the severity scale, the range of total scores is 0 to 48. As well as the individual item and total scores, the scale provides four sub-scales.

Section A – Behavioural problems (3 items).
Section B – Impairment problems (2 items).
Section C – Symptomatic problems (4 items).
Section D – Social problems (4 items).

Because the sub-scales are made up of different numbers of item scores, the sub-scale ranges are not all the same.

Uses of HoNOS in an in-patient setting

HoNOS provides a simple and easy-to-use tool for the measurement of outcome within an acute in-patient setting. It is usual for HoNOS ratings to be carried out shortly after admission and again just prior to discharge. On each of these occasions, the rating is based on the problems experienced by that individual during the previous two weeks, the difference between the two ratings at admission and discharge thus forming the measure of outcome.

This model of using the tool does work on the presumption that the individuals' period of in-patient treatment is reasonably short. Where individuals remain in-patients for significant periods of time it would be beneficial to undertake intermediate ratings during the stay to assess the ongoing outcome and provide a measurement of trends for that individual during their stay. Charlwood et al. (1999) recommend that ratings be undertaken at or around the 90-day point (± 30 days) of an extensive stay, but many staff working on in-patient units have found it useful to make a more frequent review of progress, usually monthly. It is important to remember that carrying out a HoNOS rating in itself does not take long. Individuals who are familiar with the tool usually report that it takes about five minutes to complete (Orrell et al., 1999). What is required is a full holistic assessment of the individual, but these should be conducted as part of regular reviews of an individual's progress.

One of the aspects of using HoNOS which in-patient staff sometimes report to be difficult, is gathering sufficient information about an individual's social circumstances to be able to rate the social items of the scale, particularly items 11 and 12, soon after admission (McClelland et al., 2000). In using HoNOS as a measure of outcome, it is certainly useful if the period rated at admission reflects the period of time in the community which led up to the admission becoming a necessity, since this is presumably the period of time during which the health and/or social functioning of the individual failed to such a degree that an in-patient stay was unavoidable. Practical ways of trying to overcome this are discussed later. However, it should be remembered that undertaking and recording a multidisciplinary assessment of an individual's health and social functioning is an essential part of the admission process which enables the planning of care and maps the pathway to discharge.

HoNOS provides a useful tool for working directly with clients on the ward. Indeed, its principal use should be regarded as a measure of outcome for individual patients during their stay on the ward.

The principal rationale for any assessment of an individual's clinical problems, is to try and find ways of improving the situation for that individual. By repeating HoNOS ratings, we are providing routine measures of outcome based on the client's current clinical and social presentation. This provides the opportunity to assess whether the health and social functioning of the individual has improved. When considering this issue, it is perhaps worth remembering that two caveats were used to describe the health and social gain against which to measure outcome.

1. Improvement in mental and physical health and social functioning, over and above what could be expected without intervention.
2. Maintenance of an optimal state of health and social functioning by preventing, slowing and/or mitigating deterioration. (Wing et al., 1996: 10).

Thus, its use provides a standardised measure of progress for each client on the ward, for each of the 12 individual items as well as the four subscale scores and the total score.

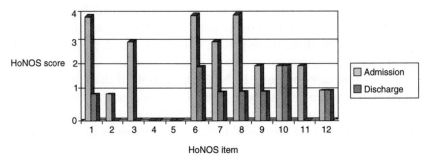

Figure 2.2 Graphical representation of HoNOS scores

It can of course be recorded as a quick checklist in an individual's clinical records, but the use of an IT system which allows the presentation of scores as a graphical output does improve the ease with which outcome for an individual can be assessed, as Figure 2.2 illustrates.

Many nurses who are routinely collecting HoNOS data report that not only is it useful in informing their own clinical work and care planning, but also that it provides a useful means of sharing information with their patients (as well as their carers) when reviewing their progress since it provides a clear focus for discussion across the 12 clinical and social items. This is of even greater value when this can be produced in a graphical format as a result of using an IT system.

Another way in which HoNOS scores can be used in routine clinical practice is to use each score as a measure of the severity of an individual's problems at that moment in time and use this as a benchmark to assess the adequacy of the current plan of care which has been devised for that individual. Each of the 12 items represents an aspect of that individual's health and social functioning, and they are all rated on the same 0 to 4 scale. Any aspect of functioning scoring a '2' or above is of clinical significance and thus should be reflected in the current plan of care. Indeed, if the planning of care for discharge from the point of admission is to be more than rhetoric, it is of particular importance that the item scores relating to the individual's social functioning are rated, since the resolution of social problems (where these exist) is often the key element in reducing the length of stay. This can prove to be a useful tool in the assessment of the quality of planned care for an in-patient population, both at an individual level and in examining a wider in-patient population. It also stresses the importance of gathering sufficient information about a client as quickly as possible after admission from as many sources as possible, particularly those in the community. It should be remembered that ratings that include '9' (no rating) cannot be used to measure outcomes either for individual items or overall scores or indeed for any of the sub-scales for which there are missing data items. Therefore, it is essential that every effort is made to collect sufficient information to make a complete rating. This may require staff to expend more time and energy on the assessment process than before, particularly in relation to contacting other professionals and agencies involved with the patient in order to build up a more comprehensive profile of the client. Time and availability of information are undoubtedly significant issues for staff in acute services. However, there is no reason why missing information cannot be entered into the rating at a later date, as long as the rater is considering the same time period (i.e., the two-week period prior to the rating). Where an incomplete rating is made, it does not mean that the HoNOS rating is totally invalid because of course the individual items that were scored can be compared, as can completed sub-sets.

The other main advantage of gathering HoNOS data is that, once aggregated and anonymised, it can, as Wing et al. (2000: 393) point out:

> provide the opportunity to measure outcome in a service-wide context where it can fulfil a vital role as a measure (not a predictor) of progress towards agreed targets and for making local comparisons.

However, HoNOS cannot be used to compare wards, districts, treatment regimes etc. unless context/background information is also collected (i.e., MDS) and like is compared with like. As the use of HoNOS becomes more widespread and its use more sophisticated then it will become possible for clinicians, managers and researchers to make more meaningful comparisons. If the HoNOS data are to be used in an aggregated form as part of a broader unit or service-wide assessment of the outcome of service populations, then its inclusion in an MDS in some form of IT system is essential. This will require, in many instances, significant investment in IT systems to ensure that the routine recording and management of data becomes possible. Experience of training mental health staff, in a variety of settings, has highlighted that access to adequate IT support systems remains far from a reality in many trusts and social service departments.

HoNOS is not directly concerned with costs or the statistics of care settings or the use of professional time (Wing et al., 1996) but it is not unreasonable for HoNOS data to be used (as part of an MDS) in the decision-making process.

Within the context of an in-patient setting, a very clear and systematic method for the use of aggregated data is set out in Severe Mental Illness Outcome Indicators (Charlwood et al., 1999). This outcome indicator is based on the principle that the aim of an acute in-patient admission is to restore the health and social functioning of those admitted and to plan discharge from this period of treatment in such a way as to minimise, as far as possible, the risk of relapse and thus the need for re-admission. It considers two elements:

1. 'Mean change in HoNOS scores, as measured on admission and discharge, within an in-patient population of people with severe mental illness';
2. 'Mean change in HoNOS scores, as measured on admission and at 90 days post admission, within an in-patient population of people with severe mental illness' (Charlwood et al., 1999: 33).

It uses all of the 12 individual item scores, as well as the four sub-scale scores and the total scores. These should be collated as

> (1) the mean differences (with associated standard deviations) in individuals' item, sub-scale and total HoNOS score, from an admission baseline to a follow-up assessment; and (2) the mean and standard deviation of the baseline scores. Item scores should be reported within their underlying range of 0–4. Subscale and total scores should be normalised to a 0–100 range. (Charlwood et al., 1999: 33)

In defining the time scales for completing these assessments, it has been assumed that the admission baseline assessment has been completed within 24 hours of admission and the discharge rating in the 24 hours immediately prior to discharge from the ward. It is also important to remember that these HoNOS data should also have additional information as part of a minimum dataset associated with it. This information will allow comparisons to be made, for example between wards or perhaps in a wider context between different provider units. Once sufficient data have been collected, they also allow comparisons to be made of the same ward over time, thus facilitating ward staff to undertake a year-on-year analysis of the global outcomes for their unit. Charlwood et al. (1999) note that if the mean changes of the data are not normally distributed, it may be more appropriate to use percentile-based statistics to undertake this outcome measurement.

Whilst this example provides clear guidance for using aggregated HoNOS data to measure outcome, this example is far from exhaustive. Indeed, it may be that the use of such a broad indicator holds limited interest to many nurses working on the wards. Only with time, fuller implementation and sharing of experiences between practitioners and services will some of the more imaginative possibilities arise. However, some further simple examples of the use of aggregated HoNOS data are provided here to help guide the thinking of individuals who aspire to using the data in their work setting.

For example, a nurse on an acute admission ward might be concerned about a rise in violent incidents on the ward and the fact that staff are finding these situations increasingly difficult to manage. Evidence from the staffing establishment provides clear evidence that there has been no change in the staff: client ratio over the preceding 12 months. Records of violent incidents will provide evidence of the increase. However, the HoNOS data could be used to provide additional information about the nature of the problem. For example, aggregated HoNOS data could identify that disability levels for the current group of clients are almost twice as high as they were six months ago with particularly high behavioural sub-scores. These three information sources would provide a clear evidence base that would usefully underpin a business case for more staff, or the creation of an Intensive Care Area, or perhaps increased funding for training in the management of violence and aggression.

Similarly, a ward manager could use aggregated HoNOS data to make a case for a member of staff to be funded for a course on substance misuse. It may be known from personal experience that a significant proportion of clients who have been admitted over the last 12 months have had a substance misuse problem but this may not have been their primary diagnosis. Using HoNOS data as part of an MDS could provide clear evidence of the scale of the problem, hence adding weight to an application for staff development money.

Wilcock (2001) provides a good example of using HoNOS data to support the planning of service development. The findings of this small-scale study indicated that female patients in a low secure in-patient setting tended to display an increase in HoNOS scores during their stay in the unit whilst male patients showed a decrease. This information was used with other information to argue a case for the development of female-only facilities.

Examining any aggregated groups of scores of a clinical area may also provide keys to areas that would benefit from further enquiry. Any set of individual scores that fail to improve over an in-patient stay would point to areas where the overall system of care may be failing to respond adequately to the needs of the clients. For example, if problems associated with non-accidental self-injury persistently lack improvement for ward populations there would be good reason to investigate these issues further, with a view to trying to improve the therapeutic interventions with clients on the ward who display these types of behaviour.

Setting-up and administration issues

From a number of years' combined experience discussing how HoNOS has been implemented in practice, one of the most important elements that appears to determine the success or otherwise of the use of HoNOS is project management. Whilst HoNOS is a simple tool in itself, developing a system of data recording and data management that meets the needs of the various groups of staff requires consideration and energy. It is not uncommon for clinical staff to receive a HoNOS pack with directions to start using it immediately. Whilst this might allow a service provider to rightly claim that they are using outcome measurement, such a strategy is fraught with dangers, the most obvious of which is that, without adequate training and ongoing supervision, the HoNOS data collected would not stand up to questions of validity and reliability (McLelland et al., 2000). In addition, staff would be unclear as to why they were using it, in what circumstances they should use it, what will happen to the data, how they can access the data to manage and monitor the caseload and so on. In many areas where inadequate thought has gone into implementation there is often a feeling of resentment and cynicism about HoNOS (and outcome measurement in general) as staff are not convinced of the clinical benefits – if staff can access the data there are few if any! It is unrealistic to expect hard-pressed staff to be overly concerned about whether the Department of Health can indicate how far services in England and Wales are meeting the goal of 'improving the health and social functioning of mentally ill people'. Staff need to see evidence of how such data can help them improve and monitor their own clinical practice and how local services are performing in the first instance.

Clear objectives have to be identified from the outset identifying the what, why, when and who of the process. All staff should sign-up to the objectives and a project team, comprising representatives of all interested parties (including the IT department), should contribute to the process. A manager who has both formal and informal authority should lead the project to ensure that agreed objectives are met, on time, to budget and of sufficient quality.

Decisions will have to be made on how HoNOS data will be recorded. Standard HoNOS score sheets are the most obvious way of gathering ratings but other methods are in use, including labels which are 'stuck' into notes and electronically, using networked or standalone computers. Whatever methods are used, clarity is needed on how this information will be entered onto the database. This sounds a rather obvious statement but frequently clinicians (and often managers) have little knowledge of what happens to HoNOS score sheets once they leave the ward or unit. In some cases they do not even do this as they are filed immediately in individual notes. Whilst this may offer some useful information for managing a particular client's programme of care it does not allow for data aggregation. There is a tendency for HoNOS data to languish in some bureaucratic 'black hole' and never see the light of day. Under such circumstances it is easy to see why many staff have become disillusioned with HoNOS; this is unfortunate since the implementation of HoNOS is clearly a useful first step in moving towards a shift in service culture towards one which is orientated around outcome measurement. Outcome measurement will not become a day-to-day reality until clinicians view it as an essential part of good practice and it is supported with adequate IT systems (Gallagher and Teesson, 2000).

It would be optimistic to believe that every Trust or Social Services Department will acquire state-of-the-art IT equipment in the short or medium term but this should not prove to be an insurmountable hurdle in implementing a data management strategy. One administrative assistant with a personal computer would be all that is needed for an organisation to store data electronically and allow staff to question the database. Obviously, giving staff direct access is preferable and this is already happening in some instances but the majority of organisations may have to work towards this ideal. Whatever the mechanism used locally, care should be taken to ensure that there are controls in place to ensure the quality and reliability of the data entered onto the system.

Training of raters and their ongoing supervision is also a major issue for organisations planning to introduce HoNOS. There are known links between the quality of training and the quality of data from the wider literature on rating scales (Ventura et al., 1993) and although HoNOS is much simpler to use than many tools, the same principles apply (Amin et al., 1999; Bebbington et al., 1999; Trauer et al., 1999). It is suggested that all potential raters undergo a structured training programme before being expected to use HoNOS routinely in clinical practice. HoNOS is undoubtedly a straightforward tool to use but there are guidelines for its use which raters have to understand and follow if HoNOS ratings are to be valid and reliable. Experience has shown that despite its simplicity misunderstandings do frequently occur when raters do not have a sufficient grasp of the basic principles of rating. In addition, it is thought that a brief one-off training course is not sufficient to guarantee comparability between individual raters or between groups of raters and that practice and ongoing supervision are required to maintain reliability and data quality.

Conclusion

As stated at the beginning of the chapter, there are numerous measures of outcome in mental health care; the debate surrounding the effective use of outcome data to inform clinical practice and service evaluation obviously extends well beyond the use of HoNOS. The brevity and comprehensive overview of functioning provided by the instrument provides a relatively easy way of embedding outcome evaluation as part-and-parcel of routine clinical practice. This is particularly important since it has the potential to link neatly with service practices and systems such as CPA, clinical governance and audit as well as inform others such as risk assessment and risk management. In addition, it can, as previously suggested, complement more specific health outcome enquiries relating to groups of service users or specific service delivery models.

It is only when mental health staff routinely record, manage and analyse outcome data against clinical intervention or service structures and delivery methods, that we will be able to say we are making rational decisions based on evidence. This will only ever represent a part of how we, as practitioners, evaluate the efficacy of the services we provide to our clients but in our opinion it is an important element. As we become more confident in our ability to use outcome data and more willing to share those experiences with our colleagues and our clients, so our decision making within both clinical practice and service planning and evaluation will become more transparent.

Resources

Website: http://www.rcpsych.ac.uk/cru/honoscales/index.htm

For general information on HoNOS (training, resources, conferences, etc.) contact: Emma George, The Royal College of Psychiatrists' Research Unit, 6th Floor, 83 Victoria Street, London SW1H 0HW.
Tel.: 020 7227 0825   Fax: 020 7227 0850   E-mail: egeorge@cru.rcpsych.ac.uk

The HoNOS Users' Forum (HUF) is for all mental health professionals using HoNOS. HUF provides an opportunity to share information and ideas about HoNOS and its use in everyday practice. Membership is free and consists of a network and a newsletter. Contact Emma George at The Royal College of Psychiatrists' Research Unit for information about membership.

Information about the work of the National Centre for Health Outcomes Development, including the work on Severe Mental Illness, can be found at http://www.ihs.ox.ac.uk

Further information about the Mental Health Information Strategy, Mental Health Minimum Data Set and other related topics can be viewed at the Department of Health website (http://www.doh.gov.uk) and the NHS Information Authority site (http://www.nhsia.nhs.uk).

Acknowledgements

Parts of this chapter are reproduced with the kind permission of the Royal College of Psychiatrists' Research Unit.

References

Amin, S., Singh, S.P., Croudace, T., Medley, I. and Harrison, G. (1999) 'Evaluating the Health of the Nation Outcome Scales. Reliability and validity in a three-year follow-up of first-onset psychosis', *British Journal of Psychiatry*, 174: 399–403.

Bebbington, P., Brugha, T., Hill, T., Marsden, L. and Window, S. (1999) 'Validation of the Health of the Nation Outcome Scales', *British Journal of Psychiatry*, 174: 389–94.

Bishop, A. (1998) *Mental Health Minimum Data Set Project: Summary Results of a Telephone Survey of Mental Health Service Providers. C3234.* London: NHS Executive.

Charlwood, P., Mason, A., Goldacre, M., Cleary, R. and Wilkinson, E. (1999) *Health Outcome Indicators: Severe Mental Illness. Report of a Working Group to the Department of Health.* Oxford: National Centre for Health Outcomes Development.

Department of Health (1992) *The Health of the Nation. A Strategy for Health in England.* London: HMSO.

Department of Health (1993) *The Health of the Nation. Key Area Handbook: Mental Health.* London: HMSO.

Department of Health (1997) *Update on the Mental Health Minimum Data Set.* London: HMSO.

Department of Health (1999) *National Service Framework for Mental Health: Modern Standards and Service Models.* London: Department of Health.

Department of Health (2001) *Mental Health Information Strategy.* London: HMSO.

Gallagher, J. and Teesson, M. (2000) 'Measuring disability, need and outcome in Australian community mental health services', *Australian and New Zealand Journal of Psychiatry*, 34 (5): 850–5.

James, M. (2002) 'The use of the Health of the Nation Outcome Scales [HoNOS] in routine clinical practice by NHS mental health service providers in England: a summary of findings', *The Approach*, 23: 13–16.

James, M. and Kehoe, R. (1999) 'Using the Health of the Nation Outcome Scales in clinical practice', *Psychiatric Bulletin*, 23 (9): 536–8.

McClelland, R., Trimble, P., Fox, M.L., Stevenson, M.R and Bell, B. (2000) 'Validation of an outcome scale for use in adult psychiatric practice', *Quality in Health Care*, 9 (2): 98–105.

NHS Information Authority (2000) *Mental Health Minimum Data Set: An Overview.* Birmingham: NHS Information Authority.

Orrell, M., Yard, P., Handysides, J. and Schapira, R. (1999) 'Validity and reliability of the Health of the Nation Outcome Scales in psychiatric patients in the community', *British Journal of Psychiatry*, 174: 409–12.

Secretary of State (1998) *Information for Health.* Wetherby: Department of Health.

Steadman, T., Yellowlees, P., Mellsop, G., Clarke, R. and Drake, S. (1997) *Measuring Consumer Outcomes in Mental Health.* Canberra: Department of Health and Family Services.

Thornicroft, G. and Tansella, M. (1996) *Mental Health Outcome Measures.* Berlin: Springer.

Trauer, T., Callaly, P., Hantz, P., Little, J., Shields, R. and Smith, J. (1999) 'Health of the Nation Outcome Scales. Results of the Victorian field trial', *British Journal of Psychiatry*, 174: 8.

Ventura, J., Green, M.F., Shaner, A. and Liberman, R.P. (1993) 'Training and quality assurance with the Brief Psychiatric Rating Scale: "The Drift Busters"', *International Journal of Methods in Psychiatric Research*, 3: 221–44.

Wilcock, A. (2001) 'The use of HoNOS in a low secure in-patient setting', *HoNOS Users' Forum Newsletter*, Autumn: 5–6.

Wing, J.K., Curtis, R.H. and Beevor, A.S. (1996) *HoNOS: Health of the Nation Outcome Scales: Report on Research and Development July 1993–December 1995*. London: Royal College of Psychiatrists.

Wing, J.K., Lelliott, P. and Beevor, A.S. (2000) 'Progress on HoNOS', *British Journal of Psychiatry*, 176: 392–3.

Further reading

Adams, M., Palmer, A., O'Brien, J.T. and Crook, W. (2000) 'Health of the Nation Outcome Scales for psychiatry: are they valid?', *Journal of Mental Health*, 9 (2): 193–8.

Allan, S. and McGonagle, I. (1997) 'A comparison of HoNOS with the Social Behaviour Schedule in three settings', *Journal of Mental Health*, 6 (2): 117–24.

Audin, K., Margison, F.R., Clark, J.M. and Barkham, M. (2001) 'Value of HoNOS in assessing patient change in NHS psychotherapy and psychological treatment services', *British Journal of Psychiatry*, 178: 561–6.

Bagley, H., Cordingley, L., Burns, A., Mozley, C.G., Sutcliffe, C., Challis, D. and Huxley, P. (2000) 'Recognition of depression by staff in nursing and residential homes', *Journal of Clinical Nursing*, 9 (3): 445–50.

Boot, B., Hall, W. and Andrews, G. (1997) 'Disability, outcome and case-mix in acute psychiatric in-patient units.', *British Journal of Psychiatry*, 171: 242–6.

British Journal of Psychiatry (2000) 'HoNOS update', *British Journal of Psychiatry*, 176: 392–5.

Brooker, C., Molyneux, P., Deverill, M. and Repper, J. (1997) 'An audit of costs and outcome using HoNOS-3 in a rehabilitation team: a pilot study', *Journal of Mental Health*, 6 (5): 491–502.

Brooker, C., Molyneux, P., Deverill, M. and Repper, J. (1999) 'Evaluating clinical outcome and staff morale in a rehabilitation team for people with serious mental health problems', *Journal of Advanced Nursing*, 29 (1): 44–51.

Brooks, R. (2000) 'The reliability and validity of the Health of the Nation Outcome Scales: validation in relation to patient derived measures', *Australian and New Zealand Journal of Psychiatry*, 34 (3): 504–11.

Browne, S., Doran, M., and McGauran, S. (2000) 'Health of the Nation Outcome Scales (HoNOS): use in an Irish psychiatric outpatient population', *Irish Journal of Psychological Medicine*, 17 (1): 17–19.

Bruce, J., Watson, D., van Teijlingen, E.R., Lawton, K., Watson, M.S. and Palin, A.N. (1999) 'Dedicated psychiatric care within general practice: health outcome and service providers' views', *Journal of Advanced Nursing*, 29 (5): 1060–7.

Burns, A., Beevor, A., Lelliott, P., Wing, J., Blakey, A., Orrell, M., Mulinga, J. and Hadden, S. (1999) 'Health of the Nation Outcome Scales for elderly people (HoNOS 65+). Glossary for HoNOS65+ score sheet', *British Journal of Psychiatry*, 174: 435–8.

Carlisle, D. (1996) 'Economies of scales', *Nursing Times*, 92 (50): 38–9.

Chaplin, R. and Perkins, R. (1999) 'HoNOS: a cautionary tale of their use in rehabilitation', *Psychiatric Bulletin*, 23 (1): 20–1.

Culiford, L., Goff-Beardsley, S. and Atkinson, T. (1999) 'Usefulness of HoNOS', *Psychiatric Bulletin*, 23 (9): 571.

Elphick, M., Anthony, P., Lines, C. and Evans, H. (1997) *Mental Health: Casemix Outcome Resource Needs: Summary Report*. Winchester: National Casemix Office.

Gilbody, S.M., House, A.O., and Sheldon, T.A. (2002) 'Psychiatrists in the UK do not use outcome measures: national survey', *Psychiatric Bulletin*, 180 (2): 101–3.

Goldney, R.D., Fisher, L.J. and Walmsley, S.H. (1998) 'The Health of the Nation Outcome Scales in psychiatric hospitalisation: a multi-centre study examining outcome and prediction of length of stay', *Australian and New Zealand Journal of Psychiatry*, 32 (2): 199–205.

Gowers, S.G., Harrington, R.C., Whitton, A., Lelliott, P., Beevor, A., Wing, J. and Jezzard, R. (1999): 'Brief scale for measuring the outcomes of emotional and behavioural disorders in children. Health of the Nation Outcome Scales for Children and Adolescents (HoNOSCA)', *British Journal of Psychiatry*, 174: 413–16.

Gowers, S.G., Harrington, R.C., Whitton, A., Beevor, A., Lelliott, P., Jezzard, R. and Wing, J.K. (1999) 'Health of the Nation Outcome Scales for Children and Adolescents (HoNOSCA): glossary for HoNOSCA score sheet', *British Journal of Psychiatry*, 174: 428–31.

Grant, B. and Deaney, C. (1998) 'Inner-city general practice population of people with schizophrenia', *Psychiatric Bulletin*, 22 (4): 221–5.

Hatfield, B., Spurrell, M. and Perry, A. (2000) 'Emergency referrals to an acute psychiatric service: demographic, social and clinical characteristics and comparisons with those receiving continuing services', *Journal of Mental Health*, 9 (3): 305–17.

Hugo, M., Smout, M. and Bannister, J. (2002) 'A comparison in hospitalisation rates between a community-based mobile emergency service and a hospital-based emergency service', *Australian and New Zealand Journal of Psychiatry*, 36 (4): 504–8.

Issakidis, C. and Teesson, M. (1999) 'Measurement of need for care: a trial of the Camberwell Assessment of Need and the Health of the Nation Outcome Scales', *Australian and New Zealand Journal of Psychiatry*, 33 (5): 754–9.

Jeffries, M. (1996) 'A culture of effective efficiency', *NHS Magazine*, 6: 12–13.

Lambert, G., Caputi, P. and Deane, F.P. (2002) 'Sources of information when rating using the Health of the Nation Outcome Scales', *International Journal of Mental Health Nursing*, 11: 135–8.

McEvoy, P., Colgan, S. and Richards, D. (2002) 'Gatekeeping access to community mental health teams: differences in practice between consultant psychiatrists, senior house officers and community psychiatric nurses', *Psychiatric Bulletin*, 26 (2): 56–8.

Milne, D., Reichelt, K. and Wood, E. (2001) 'Implementing HoNOS: an eight stage approach', *Clinical Psychology and Psychotherapy*, 8: 106–16.

Page, A., Hooke, G. and Rutherford, E. (2001) 'Measuring mental health outcomes in a private psychiatric clinic: Health of the Nation Outcome Scales and Medical Outcomes Short Form SF-36', *Australian and New Zealand Journal of Psychiatry*, 35 (3): 377–81.

Parker, G., O'Donnell, M., Hadzi-Pavlovic, D. and Proberts, M. (2002) 'Assessing outcome in community mental health patients: a comparative analysis of measures', *International Journal of Social Psychiatry*, 48 (1): 11–19.

Pirkis, J., Burgess, P. and Jolley, D. (1999) 'Suicide attempts by psychiatric patients in acute inpatient, long-stay inpatient and community care', *Social Psychiatry and Psychiatric Epidemiology*, 34 (12): 634–44.

Preston, N.J. (2000) 'The Health of the Nation Outcome Scales: validating factorial structure and invariance across two health services', *Australian and New Zealand Journal of Psychiatry*, 34 (3): 512–19.

Rock, D. and Preston, N. (2001) 'HoNOS: is there any point in training clinicians?', *Journal of Psychiatric and Mental Health Nursing*, 8: 405–9.

Roy, A., Matthews, H., Clifford, P., Fowler, V. and Martin, M.M. (2002) 'Health of the Nation Outcome Scale for People with Learning Disabilities (HoNOS-LD)', *British Journal of Psychiatry*, 180: 61–70.

Rushforth, D., Brooker, C., Winstanley, J. and Repper, D. (2000) 'The use of HoNOS in the evaluation of partial hospitalisation in mental health day care ... Health of the Nation Outcome Scales', *Clinical Effectiveness in Nursing*, 4 (3): 121–7.

Sharma, V.K., Wilkinson, G. and Fear, S. (1999) 'Health of the Nation Outcome Scales: a case study in general psychiatry', *British Journal of Psychiatry*, 174: 395–8.

Slade, M., Beck, A., Bindman, J., Thornicroft, G. and Wright, S. (1999) 'Routine clinical outcome measures for patients with severe mental illness: CANSAS and HoNOS', *British Journal of Psychiatry*, 174: 404–8.

Taylor, J.R. and Wilkinson, G. (1997) 'HoNOS vs opinion in a shifted out-patient clinic', *Psychiatric Bulletin*, 21 (8): 483–5.

Trauer, T. (1999) 'The subscale structure of the Health of the Nation Outcome Scales (HoNOS)', *Journal of Mental Health*, 8 (5): 499–509.

Trauer, T. and Callaly, T. (2002) 'Concordance between patients and their case managers using Health of the Nation Outcome Scales (HoNOS)', *Australasian Psychiatry*, 10 (1): 24–8.

Trauer, T., Callaly, T. and Hantz, P. (1999) 'The measurement of improvement during hospitalisation for acute psychiatric illness', *Australian and New Zealand Journal of Psychiatry*, 33 (3): 379–84.

Wing, J.K., Curtis, R.H. and Beevor, A. (1999) 'Health of the Nation Outcome Scales (HoNOS): glossary for HoNOS score sheet', *British Journal of Psychiatry*, 174: 432–4.

Wing, J., Lelliott, P. and Chaplin, R.H. (1999) 'Reliability and validity of HoNOS (multiple letters)', *Psychiatric Bulletin*, 23 (6): 375.

Wing, J.K., Beevor, A., Curtis, R.H., Park, S.B.G., Hadden, S. and Burns, A. (1998) 'Health of the Nation Outcome Scales (HoNOS): research and development', *British Journal of Psychiatry*, 172: 11–18.

THREE

Social inclusion and acute care

Julie Repper and Rachel Perkins

Introduction

The idea of 'social inclusion' is often not considered in relation to 'acute care'. Whereas social inclusion is about social roles, networks, relationships and community, acute care is about treatment in a crisis, sometimes requiring time away from social roles and relationships. However, if a person's social roles, networks and relationships are to be maintained over periods of acute crisis, social inclusion must be high on the agenda during periods of acute psychiatric in-patient care.

Acute episodes of mental distress can jeopardise social inclusion by disrupting family relationships, friendships, social networks, employment and social/leisure activities. A person may behave in uncharacteristic ways that are disturbing to others. They may become unable to meet the expectations of their social, work and leisure roles. If a person attempts to continue with their ordinary social roles when they are unable to fulfil them, then it is likely that these roles will be disrupted. In such a situation, a period of admission to an acute psychiatric ward may be positively beneficial in maintaining a person's social roles by relieving them of responsibilities and expectations that they are temporarily unable to fulfil.

However, it is often the case that far from assisting in the preservation of social roles and relationships, psychiatric admission can further erode them to the point where the person has access only to the devalued role of the patient. If social roles and relationships are to be preserved through a period of admission, it is essential that acute in-patient services actively attend to the maintenance of a person's social roles and relationships during a period of admission and help the person to resume their ordinary roles as the admission nears its end (Rose, 2001). This involves both assisting the person to keep in touch with those people who are important to them – family, friends, employers, others in their social network – and supporting these other people and agencies as appropriate so that the person is able to return when they are well enough to do so.

This chapter begins by considering social inclusion, and the exclusion that so often accompanies the experience of mental health problems and the use of mental health services. It then goes on to examine the experience of admission to an acute psychiatric ward and its impact upon the individual, their family and their friends, and others who are important in the person's social world like employers, colleagues, teachers. Finally, ways in which positive, socially inclusive strategies can be fostered on acute wards are considered in order to minimise the social disruption and damage that admission so often causes, and to use the opportunity to strengthen existing relationships and/or initiate new roles. The chapter draws on examples of good practice to explore the development and outcome of socially inclusive ways of working in acute in-patient settings.

What is social inclusion?

There is considerable evidence to suggest that people with mental health problems experience significant discrimination in their daily lives. Individuals who experience mental health problems are being systematically excluded from many areas of society, including employment and training, access to services and many other areas of daily living. The accounts of those who have experienced mental health problems provide testimony to the exclusion from the roles and relationships that the rest of us take for granted and their rejection when applying for training, jobs and insurance (Dunn, 1999). Read and Baker (1996) revealed the extent of this discrimination and exclusion in the findings of a survey of 778 people who had experienced mental distress:

- 34% had been dismissed or forced to resign from jobs;
- 69% had been put off applying for jobs for fear of unfair treatment;
- 47% had been abused or harassed in public (11% had been physically attacked) and 26% had been forced to move home because of harassment;
- 50% felt they had been unfairly treated by physical health services;
- 33% complained that their GP had treated them unfairly;
- 25% had been turned down by insurance or finance companies.

Too often, the views, accounts and experiences of someone who experiences mental health difficulties are taken to be simply a manifestation of these difficulties:

I can speak but I may not be heard. I can make suggestions, but they may not be taken seriously. I can voice my thoughts, but they may be seen as delusions. I can recite experiences, but they may be interpreted as fantasies. To be a patient or even an ex-patient is to be discounted. (Leete, 1988: 2)

The process of social exclusion has been defined by the government's Social Exclusion Unit as:

A shorthand for what can happen when individuals or areas suffer from a combination of linked problems such as unemployment, poor skills, low incomes, poor housing, high crime environments, bad health and family breakdown. (Social Exclusion Unit, 1999)

This process is not surprising in a society where there is a general perception that mental health problems are inevitably associated with dangerousness and/or incompetence. Dunn (1999) and Sayce (2000) have described how those who experience mental health problems are among the most excluded in society. Discrimination against them is one of the last 'acceptable' prejudices effectively denying citizenship. Sayce gives an account of how social exclusion develops and affects people with mental health problems, through a combination of overlapping problems including mental impairment, discrimination, reduced social and economic participation, diminishing hope and expectations (Sayce, 2000).

This account epitomises the complexity of the relationship between mental health and social exclusion: exclusion can both lead to mental health problems and be a consequence of them. For example, unemployment leads to an increase in the risk of mental health problems (Smith, 1985; Warr, 1987). Yet pervasive employment discrimination ensures that the experience of mental health problems is also a cause of unemployment: unemployment can both lead to mental health problems and be a consequence of them. The 1997/98 *Labour Force Survey* revealed that unemployment among those with mental health problems is alarmingly high at 87%, far higher than among disabled people more generally (Burchardt, 2000).

What is clear, however, is that for all the high hopes of 'community care', exclusion of the mentally ill is not decreasing. Department of Health surveys show that the proportion of people expressing fear of people with mental health problems has risen: in 1993, 14% of a representative sample of adults thought it was frightening to think of people with mental health problems living in residential areas; this figure rose to 19% in 1996 and 25% in 1997 (DoH, 1997). As Campbell (2000: 88) has observed:

The great irony about service user action in the past 15 years is that, while the position of service users within services has undoubtedly improved, the position of service users in society has deteriorated.

Although 'community care' appeared to carry the potential for people with mental health problems to be integrated in mainstream society, they remain as firmly excluded today as they ever were behind the walls of the asylum.

The importance of action to maintain and improve social inclusion is evident in all recent mental health policy and is enshrined in Standard 1 of the National Service Framework (DoH, 1999a), which states that services must

> combat discrimination against individuals and groups with mental health problems and promote their social inclusion.

Similarly, both the Mental Health Promotion Strategy (DoH, 2000b) and the National Service Framework (DoH, 1999a), specify the need to include employment and housing plans in Care Programme Approach care plans, and job retention schemes for people with mental health problems have been the subject of a large DfEE-funded research scheme.

Promoting social inclusion must be a primary concern to mental health workers. The development of strategies to enable people to maintain and develop those social roles, relationships, networks and activities that are central to social inclusion is the responsibility of all mental health practitioners. Such endeavours cannot be limited to those working in community services. Admission to acute in-patient settings can easily increase discrimination and exclusion. If such admissions are to be beneficial in maintaining a person's social roles then attention to the maintenance and extension of these must also be a central component of work in in-patient settings.

Social exclusion in acute care settings

The impact of admission of the individual

The experience of acute mental distress is often traumatic enough in itself. People who have been through it have written numerous accounts of the extremes of emotion, unfamiliarity of beliefs and feelings, difficulty controlling behaviours and unpredictability of others' responses (see Read, 1996). Admission to an acute ward can compound these problems, but it also heralds many more difficulties through the reactions of others – because of the irrefutable stigma that time 'inside the madhouse' brings.

Whilst admission is designed to provide 'asylum', respite, safety, careful assessment and treatment, this is often not the experience of the recipient. Already frightened by the experience of acute crisis, the experience of admission can compound these problems. As long ago as 1989, Camden Mental

Health Consortium (GPMH, 1989) described the deleterious consequences of admission, and the Sainsbury Centre for Mental Health (2000) has documented the ways in which care provided on acute units continues to be inadequate. Such wards are often experienced as unsafe, unclean, unpredictable, untherapeutic places where staff have little time to spend with residents and there is a dearth of explanation, choice, treatment (other than medication) and little to do (as described in earlier chapters: SNMAC, 1999; SCMH, 2000; Mind, 2001) – hardly a place to 'get better'.

Although service users frequently comment on the helpfulness of individual members of staff (see Chadwick, 1996), their accounts portray a system dominated by medication and containment in which they are considered unfit to make responsible decisions, unlikely to recover and disconnected from social networks, social routines and social responsibilities (see 'Real lives: the acute ward experience', Sainsbury Centre for Mental Health, 2000: 29).

Admission and friends

The experience of acute mental distress and admission impacts not only on the individual who experiences them, but also on those around them. In a survey of 421 friends of people experiencing mental distress, the Mental Health Foundation (2001) found that a number of people felt powerless and helpless, 'not knowing how to cope with the effects'. This is particularly marked when a friend is admitted to hospital, with accounts describing feelings of shock and worry at conditions within mental health units but also fear associated with mental illness. These types of responses are not surprising in a society where media representations of people with mental health problems are almost universally negative. This situation is compounded by a chronic absence of a user voice in the media (Sayce, 2000).

Despite ample evidence to the contrary, the media continue to present an alarming picture of 'a rising tide of killings' by people with mental health problems. Philo et al. (1993) found that two-thirds of media coverage of mental health issues focused on violent behaviour – a trend that is on the increase (Muijen, 1997). On top of its direct effect upon the individual, admission marks a difference in the nature of relationships with family and friends. It confirms their madness: what might have been perceived as difference, eccentricity, normal distress, now becomes recognised as mental illness – medically, and therefore socially, validated. Friends and family feel unsure how to relate to this person they may have known for many years – and this adds to the difficulties of those experiencing mental health problems.

Unsurprisingly, friends are as important to people with mental health problems as they are for all of us. In the Mental Health Foundation survey, 367 people with mental health problems described their relationships:

80% described emotional support from friends – understanding, accepting, listening, talking – and 46% reported friends providing practical support such as help with household chores, transport to appointments and financial support. Yet, such social support is disrupted by admission to hospital. In a study of 310 people with mental health problems, Holmes-Eber and Riger (1990) found that lengthy and repeated admissions were associated with smaller social networks comprising fewer friends and relatives and more professionals and fellow service users, whilst people who had been admitted less often and for shorter time periods had more friends and fewer mental health professionals in their networks.

Holmes-Eber and Riger (1990) argue that these findings provide a good case for reducing psychiatric hospital admissions to a minimum. Yet, although developments in community care and home treatment can reduce the need for admission, there is no evidence that such admissions can be eliminated completely. Therefore it is equally important that social relationships be supported during hospital admissions: friends should be recognised as an important source of support. In the Mental Health Foundation survey of friends, 58% of friends wanted support in giving their friends support. They cited the kinds of support that would be useful as:

- talking to a professional (39%);
- more information (27%);
- information about their friend's care (23%);
- time out from their friend (21%).

Admission and the family

Families play an important role in the lives of many people with mental health problems: they are an important resource and often central in the promotion and maintenance of social inclusion. They:

- enable people to retain links with their local community;
- provide important social contacts for people whose social networks are often depleted as a result of their mental health problems;
- provide a great deal of ongoing support that people need and an environment in which they can recover (Kuipers, 2001).

However, the difficulties which relatives experience have also been widely documented (e.g., Creer et al., 1982; Fadden et al., 1987). Living with someone with serious ongoing mental health problems can cause increased strain, worry and distress, together with loss of friends and social contacts, social isolation and difficulties in coping with particular symptoms.

The National Service Framework (DoH, 1999a) and the Carers' Strategy (DoH, 1999c) explicitly recognise the role that relatives play and prioritise their needs. Appleby (2000), the National Director of Mental Health, accords families a central place in defining a high-quality mental health service, recognising their skills as carers and arguing for their place in routine care planning. However, while the experiences and needs of relatives have received more attention than those of friends, families continue to fight to be heard (see Rethink (www.rethink.org) for examples). It is widely recognised that family members need respite, emotional support, practical help and information, but it remains the case that services have great difficulty in providing these things. Relatives often feel relatively ill-informed and unsupported by staff who do not recognise the contribution they make, and the difficulties they experience, and feel that staff blame them for their relative's problems (Shepherd et al., 1995).

It is often during admission that they feel most distressed, excluded and powerless. Admission of a family member is stigmatising and families have to overcome the prejudices and misconceptions of those around them. As this account shows, the stigma of mental illness – and of using mental health services – can lead family members to be socially excluded, or to exclude themselves:

> I became involved in the world of mental illness [25 years ago] … Then, I thought that mental illness couldn't happen to my family. It was something that happened to 'weak' people. I still have people asking me at the dinner table, 'is it catching?' They ask these questions because they fear mental illness. There is a great deal of shame attached to severe mental illness. Carers fear loss of face, lowering of standards, *the shame of attending or visiting psychiatric hospital* and perhaps admitting to not being able to cope. (Fisher, 2003 [Chairman, 'Rethink', 2003] in introduction to 'Rethink' website; emphasis added).

Families provide the bulk of support for people who have mental health problems (Rethink estimate that 70% of all care is provided by informal carers, with a value of £30 million per year). They are often strong advocates for individuals who have mental health problems, fighting for the best support available. They need and deserve support and recognition from services, particularly when they are likely to be most distressed – when their relative is admitted to an acute ward. Yet, not infrequently acute distress is associated with a rift in family relationships, and the individual admitted may object to their family being involved in their care in any way.

This places staff in a difficult position: how to accede to the wishes of the individual and gain their trust as well as meeting the needs of, and involving, relatives (Winefield and Burnett, 1996). The practitioner is obliged to respect a service user's wish not to involve their relatives, or provide them with information about the care that they are receiving (unless the family has been appointed by a court to manage the individual's affairs, or if there is a 'public interest' reason for giving them information). This can cause further difficulties in family relationships, leading relatives to feel excluded and ill-informed. However, concerns about confidentiality must not be used as an excuse for ignoring carers. The National Service Framework for Mental Health (DoH, 1999a) requires that relatives have access to services in their own right. It is possible to take seriously and address the concerns of both the service user and their relatives without breaching confidentiality. Nevertheless, situations where the wishes of an individual and their family differ can make the practitioner feel obliged to 'side' with one or other party. Such situations may arise around issues relating to mental health problems and medication, but also around concerns outside the psychiatric sphere. For example, such differences not uncommonly arise around the ordinary developmental issues that challenge most families in late adolescence like sex, drink, drugs and what constitutes 'acceptable' behaviour. Staff may feel torn between the wishes of the relative and those of the service user. However, this does not rule out the possibility of empathising with the positions of both parties and helping them to work out a mutually tolerable way forward – but this requires time and expertise that may not be available to the practitioner. Therefore staff training in working with families, and the allocation of time and ongoing supervision to ensure that this training can be used in practice, are essential.

It is often the case that crises in family relationships are temporary: understandable resentment about family involvement in an involuntary admission, paranoid ideas about family members and mutual mistrust generally abate, and the individual who lived with their family up to admission is likely to return to live with their family. Therefore, preserving and enhancing relationships with families during an in-patient stay is important.

Admission and colleagues, employers and neighbours

Reciprocal affection and support developed over long periods of time are characteristic of relationships with family and close friends, and this can mean that all parties are highly motivated to try to maintain relationships during a crisis. However, less intimate relationships with neighbours, colleagues, employers, more distant relatives and other social contacts are equally important in the lives of most people and much more readily lost as a result of mental health crisis and admission.

People in the individual's community are often afraid of what mental illness means. They may be shocked that someone on their street could have mental illness, unwilling to be seen in the company of someone with this affliction, may simply ignore that individual (and their family) – effectively withdrawing support and, through ostracisation, making their life more difficult. Barham and Hayward (1995) have described how people make efforts to 'prove' their 'sanity' and trustworthiness to friends and neighbours following acute relapse.

Employment has long been acknowledged as central to social inclusion (Bennett, 1975). Work links an individual to the society in which they live: without work, these links are all too easily lost – a fact recognised in various government 'New Deal' policies, including the New Deal for Disabled People which explicitly includes those with mental health problems. As well as an income, work provides social identity and status; social contacts and support; a means of structuring and occupying time; activity and involvement; and a sense of personal achievement (Jahoda et al., 1933; Bennett, 1975; Shepherd, 1984; Warr, 1987; Rowland and Perkins, 1988; Pozner et al., 1996; Grove, 1999). Work tells us who we are and enables us to tell others who we are: it is typically the second question we ask when we meet someone: 'What is your name?', 'What do you do?'

The existence of work in a person's life is a necessary counterpoint to leisure: without work – the things we have to do – the concept of leisure – free time – is meaningless (Rowland and Perkins, 1988). Jahoda et al. (1933) showed that unemployed people do not exploit the extra time they have available for leisure and social pursuits. Their social networks and social functioning decrease, as do motivation and interest, leading to apathy.

A person's employment is severely jeopardised by acute mental health crisis and admission. At first admission many people are in employment. Yet many employers are reluctant to retain, or take on, employees with mental health problems, the prevailing stereotypes of mental illness causing them to believe that workers with such difficulties are likely to be dangerous, unreliable, unpredictable, unproductive. Many people who are admitted to hospital may have behaved inappropriately at work prior to admission and even a sympathetic employer may not know what to do to help. Therefore contact with, and support for, employers is essential if people are to be able to return to their employment on discharge. For those in education, the role of the student is equally important, but teachers and lecturers may share much of the ignorance and prejudice of employers and fail to make the adjustments necessary to enable the person to resume their course once they are discharged. Again contact with and support for education providers is equally important in maintaining a person's social inclusion.

Once on an acute ward, social roles, activities and routines are suspended, family relationships are disrupted, time is taken off work or college, and friends are rarely encouraged to visit. On discharge, the individual has the stressful task of picking up old activities; re-establishing family relationships; explaining their absence to work colleagues, teachers and classmates; and re-establishing old friendships. This is doubly difficult as they have to battle against the misconceptions, mistrust and fear associated with 'madness' in general, while trying to demonstrate their own ability at the same time as trying to accommodate into their lives the mental health problems they have experienced. Without the maintenance of links with the outside world during an in-patient stay, appropriate preparation to resume social roles on discharge, and ongoing support in the community, many people find this challenge too daunting. They therefore fail to resume their former social roles and social exclusion results. If this is to be avoided, social inclusion must be central to the work of acute in-patient settings.

Social inclusion in acute settings

An inclusive philosophy

Developing a 'philosophy of care' can seem an irrelevant diversion on a busy acute ward: a gesture, resulting in nothing more than a sign on the wall that is regarded with cynicism by staff and patients alike. However, it is essential for the whole team to be clear about what they are working towards, how they are working and what values underpin their work. This philosophy needs to be worked out as a team, differences between members of staff need to be acknowledged (they are unlikely to be overcome) and implications for practice need to be explored.

The philosophy and priorities of an acute in-patient setting are central in maintaining and promoting the social roles, relationships and activities of those who are admitted. However, it is typically the case that the primary concerns on acute in-patient units are safety, containment and pharmacological treatment. While these may be important, they are not sufficient to maintain and promote social inclusion. If, on discharge, a person is unable to resume their former roles, relationships and activities, or develop new ones, then their mental health problems are likely to be exacerbated and the likelihood of further admissions increased. Promoting social inclusion is not only important in relation to social functioning, it is also important in maintaining and enhancing both physical and mental health. For example, unemployment has been linked with increased general health problems, including premature death (Beale and Nethercott, 1985; Smith, 1985; Bartley, 1994) and there is a particularly strong relationship between unemployment and mental health difficulties (Warr, 1987;

Warner, 1994). Unemployment is associated with increased use of mental health services (Brenner and Bartell, 1983; Wilson and Walker, 1993; Warner, 1994; Stewart, 1996) and is known to increase the risk of suicide (Platt and Kreitman, 1984; Moser et al., 1987; Philippe, 1988; Lewis and Sloggett, 1998). The absence of social supports and social networks is equally detrimental to mental health (see Simmons, 1994).

This means that, in developing a philosophy of care, acute wards must consider their role not only in alleviating symptoms, but also in preserving and developing social roles and relationships. This involves attention to both the individual and their social world. Wing and Morris (1981) have described how social disability results not only from the symptoms which someone experiences, but also from the way in which they respond to these symptoms and the discrimination that it creates.

In the face of the terrifying consequences of mental health problems and psychiatric admission on a person's life, two responses are common: the person may either 'give up' or deny that they have any difficulties (Deegan, 1993). Both of these responses jeopardise a person's social roles and relationships by making them less able to use the skills and abilities they have: either they lose hope and fail to recognise their strengths or they fail to accept the support and help they need to minimise the disruptive effect of their mental health problems (Perkins and Repper, 1996). The person's experience of acute admission is central in helping them to adapt to their mental health problems and rebuild a satisfying and valued life, and in this process hope is of the essence.

People who have survived the experience of admission to an acute ward, write of the need for hope. Too often staff who work on acute wards see people only at the point when their mental health problems are most severe. They do not see what these people can achieve between acute crises and therefore it is not surprising that expectations become tarnished. Having only a view of the individual at their most incapacitated, there is a tendency to fail to recognise their skills and abilities and be pessimistic about what they can achieve: they will never be able to work, raise children, have an 'ordinary' life. Such a perspective further destroys confidence and de-skills people and promotes a dependency and passivity that prevents people exploring what is meaningful and valuable to them, thereby hampering growth and the development of the positive sense of self necessary to enable the person to resume their social roles and relationships.

The 'hope-inspiring' competencies of staff are therefore central. It is essential that staff value every person, recognise their potential, nurture their hopes. Nothing is more likely to lead to a person giving up than a loss of hope. Routine under-estimation of a person's potential can itself be a significant contributor to 'negative symptoms' such as 'lack of motivation'.

Rather, staff can help to identify a way towards realising dreams. Thus, for example, the desire for a job will help provide the motivation for getting up, washing and dressing on a regular basis, preparing an application, practising for an interview, all of which may fuel the recovery process even if job interviews do not prove immediately successful.

But what is most important is that every member of staff examines their own attitudes towards people who have mental health problems. Do they really believe in the potential of these people? Do they respect them? Do they value them? Or do their doubts leak out into their day-to-day work? These are questions for clinical supervision, but they are also important in establishing a ward team that provides consistency, time, support, warmth and acceptance of (if not always agreement with) the people they are working with.

Gaining control over one's problems is central in promoting hope and recovery; therefore, attention needs to be given to promoting self-management of difficulties. This should involve enabling a person to monitor their own difficulties and crisis/relapse planning to reduce the destructive impact of exacerbations of their problems on their lives. If a person is able to identify problems early and take the necessary remedial action, this can decrease the disruptive effect of their problems on their lives and relationships and thus promote their social inclusion.

But as well as gaining control over mental health problems, recovery and inclusion involve enabling the person to take control over their own life. If a person is to resume their roles and relationships and rebuild their life, then it is important that acute ward staff attend to the things that are important to service users, even when these differ from what practitioners think is best for them. It is only by ascertaining what people want to achieve and helping them to achieve it that social inclusion can be promoted. Read (1996) describes the eight things that users most want as: choice; accessibility; advocacy; equal opportunities; income and employment; self-help and self-organisation. In a study of users' perceptions of their *unmet* needs, Estroff (1993) found the most common to be: an adequate income, intimacy and privacy, a satisfying sex life, meaningful work, a satisfying social life, happiness, adequate resources and warmth. The same themes were echoed in a study of what users wanted from mental health staff: better information and choice, more accessible help, and practical help with: income and benefits; finding employment; housing; daily living skills; child care; and help in accessing appropriate specialist services (Duggan et al., 1997). A series of focus groups conducted to elicit users' and carers' views of the core competencies of mental health workers emphasised values and attitudes over skills (Institute for Health Care Development, 1998). The priorities of this mixed group included: respect, optimism, ability to manage the power imbalance between users and professionals, belief in the value of a trusting relationship, ability to 'let go' of the service user, flexibility, openness and the ability to work across traditional boundaries. Similarly, Newnes (1994: 46), reporting on a series of workshops involving service users and service providers, compiled a list of factors that sustain mental health:

> Privacy, peace, quiet, physical comfort, friendship, love, freedom to participate, support, money, work, information, exercise, a sense of belonging and realistic expectation.

The philosophy of practice on an acute ward must therefore be inclusive in a number of ways.

- Inclusive of social perspective – the person's roles and relationships – as well as their symptoms.
- Inclusive of a person's strengths – and developing these – as well as alleviating their symptoms.
- Inclusive of those who are important in the person's life – family, friends, employers – and the importance of supporting the person's relationships.
- Inclusive of the way in which a person copes with the experience of mental health problems and their symptoms – and promotes the person's independence and autonomy in managing their problems.
- Inclusive of the person's own aspirations and goals – and enabling the person to take control over rebuilding their life after illness.

An inclusive environment

Whilst the extent to which the experience of acute admission promotes social inclusion depends largely on the philosophy and practices of the ward team, the physical environment is also important – for staff as well as for those who use the service (DoH, 2000a; Sainsbury Centre for Mental Health, 2000). People can only retain any self-esteem if they are respected, but all too often in-patient wards are demeaning places, which convey to their residents the message that they are not valued. Can there be anything more devaluing than to be seen as unfit to use the 'staff toilets' or use the same crockery as staff? One of the problems with psychiatric units, especially those in District General Hospitals, is that they often share the features of the medical and surgical wards in the same building. Thus they often have long corridors, linoleum floors, glass-fronted staff offices from which they can be observed, numerous internal treatment/interview rooms and stifling temperatures. The poor catering so frequently found in all NHS facilities has been the focus of much concern (DoH, 2000a). Yet, unlike medical or surgical wards, residents are not lying in beds, but often pacing up and down, sitting around the edge of institutionally furnished rooms with a television blaring forth – a far cry from the personal, warm and safe feeling conveyed by some of the crisis houses that have developed for people in mental distress (Reeves, 1999).

It is vital that the ward environment feels welcoming, not only for the individual patient but also for their relatives and friends. Many people have never been inside a psychiatric facility and retain images of 'madhouses', 'strait-jackets' and the like. If a person's social roles and relationships are to be maintained and promoted it is critical that visiting the ward is a pleasant experience, and inviting facilities for visitors, that afford some privacy, are essential. One room might be designated specifically for this purpose with comfortable chairs, pictures, access to refreshments and information packs about the unit (what it is for, who is who, the routine, answers to common questions, etc.) with additional details about the nature of mental distress, different types of support/treatment provided and alternative forms of support or therapy that might be helpful. But written information is not enough. Seeing someone you love in acute distress can be a difficult experience, and family and friends need information and support from staff when they visit. Suitable arrangements, and support, for children to visit their relatives in hospital must also be considered.

Whilst this might seem unrealistic to staff immersed in the hurly-burly of acute admission wards housed in what are essentially unsuitable environments, many changes are possible at little cost. It may not be possible to change the bricks and mortar, but it is possible to think about the way in which the space is used. Keeping bathrooms and kitchens locked, removing access to cutlery, separate staff toilets and sitting rooms, avoiding use of carpets because of the risk of cigarette burns and spillages, all derive from a dehumanising philosophy in which in-patients are neither valued nor trusted. It is not difficult to identify ways in which things can be improved – even in the barren structure of a DGH ward. Fresh flowers, rugs, bright curtains to provide privacy. Pictures, patients' own artwork, poetry, a library of books in good condition, recent magazines. Areas for women only, areas for smokers, areas where drinks and snacks can be made around the clock as patients wish. Private, comfortable visitors' facilities. For example, most in-patient areas have a room – often an area currently used by staff: a doctor's room, interview room or staff sitting room – that could be transformed into space for visitors. A lot can be achieved with a little creativity and ingenuity.

Inclusive practices

An inclusive philosophy and environment are of little value unless they are matched by socially inclusive practices. In this context inclusion is important in relation to the people who are admitted to the ward, and their relatives and friends, as well as employers, lecturers and other social contacts.

Including service users

Socially inclusive practices must start with the inclusion of service users.

- Inclusion at all levels of service provision, from the planning and delivery of individual care, through the operation of the individual ward, and the monitoring and evaluation of services to service planning and development (Health Advisory Service, 1999).
- A recognition of the value of service users as citizens and their role within our communities and their rights to those things that most people take for granted: information, choice, respect, dignity, a decent place to live, a decent income, a job. Access to the roles, relationships and activities that non-disabled citizens enjoy: social contacts and supports.

Information and involvement in the planning and delivery of individual care are paramount in enhancing outcomes and satisfaction and promoting engagement with services (Wallcraft, 1994). Attention should be paid to the mechanisms employed to facilitate such involvement. The 'ward round' can be a terrifying place and few people would be comfortable talking about personal matters in a room full of professionals, many of whom they knew only vaguely, if at all. People on acute wards may find it difficult to express their views, both because of their mental health problems and the nature of the situation they are in. Read (1996) suggests that whilst professionals may not see themselves as intimidating, the nature of the relationship is often such that people feel constrained about what they can say, particularly when they believe it is not what professionals want to hear.

The presence of someone whom the person knows and trusts may help them to express their wishes and concerns. This may be a friend or relative (many of us find the support of a friend or relative important in attending a doctor's appointment), but access to independent advocacy may also be important. Sometimes staff feel threatened by the presence of a friend or advocate, but this is a mistake. As Leader and Crosby (1998) argue, advocacy has a central role to play in improving genuine partnership working between service users and mental health workers. However, advocacy should not be limited to care planning within services.

As well as individual treatment and support, involvement must also extend to the operation of the ward and the practices that are adopted. Inclusion should involve, for example, staff and residents eating meals together, using the same toilets and crockery and an opportunity to have an input into the operation of the ward, as well as into staff training and selection and the development of services. The 'expertise of experience' should also be included in the staff team by the recruitment of people who have themselves experienced mental health problems (see Perkins, 1998). If social inclusion is to be promoted in a wider social context, it must also be promoted within psychiatric services themselves.

Such involvement is enshrined in all recent government policy and is straightforward when practitioner and client agree. However, the views of staff and clients can differ (Dimsdale et al., 1979; Shepherd et al., 1995) and this poses challenges for staff. Although there are some constraints on choice, like those relating to compulsory detention, this does not preclude involvement completely; however, it does challenge the prevailing assumption that the 'professional knows best'.

The challenge for the acute ward team is to develop ways of working that ensure that people have as much choice in the care they receive as is possible. To promote a culture and ways of working that ensure all people on the ward are listened to, trusted, believed in, acknowledged as experts in their own experiences, allowed to set their own goals and make their own choices wherever possible (for some this might be limited to enabling them to determine when to get up, what to wear, what to eat and where to sit) – and respecting those choices even if not agreeing. The focus of care needs to rest on assets and abilities rather than deficits and difficulties. Service users typically see their problems arising within the context of their lives as a whole, and they only want to address these symptoms if, and to the extent that, they prevent them from accessing other aspects of their lives (see Repper, 2000).

A social inclusion agenda requires acute wards to address the individual in the context of their life: those roles, relationships and activities that are important to the person. This involves extending the remit of assessment and intervention beyond symptomatology:

> ... just as diagnosis is only one part of a person's life, so medical treatment is only one part of the support they need – to cope, to recover and to avoid relapse. The other support – by far the largest part – will come from family, friends, schools, employers, faith communities, neighbourhoods – and from opportunities to enjoy the same range of services and facilities within the community as everyone else. (DoH, 2000b: 45)

The first step must be to ascertain the roles, relationships and activities that are important to the person. We need to ask people about family members and friends to whom they may be particularly close; whether they have a job; whether there are other people – neighbours, religious leaders, people from the football team in which the person plays or the self-help group of which they are a part – that the person is in contact with. It is only by knowing about the person's social contacts, roles and networks that we can hope to help the person to maintain these over the period of admission.

Including family and friends

Although staff in acute settings generally aim to involve family members, this is often done on an impromptu basis, rarely afforded priority in the urgency of admission, and more frequently done in response to requests from the family. Staff often have little training or ongoing support in working with families (Fadden, 1997). Certainly families and friends do not feel adequately involved: they do not feel that their accounts are heeded, and their own needs are often unmet. Whilst plans to keep the family informed of progress and treatment are often intended, these will only be implemented effectively if a clear system of support and involvement of family and friends is planned and agreed by the whole team and implemented throughout the entire admission period.

The National Carers Strategy (DoH, 1999c: see www.doh.gov.uk/carers/pdfs) is a useful resource for ward teams seeking to develop a strategy to involve carers. It reviews the important role that carers play, their views on services and their needs, and it outlines government initiatives to support carers. Although not specific to mental health, it clarifies legislation and gives examples of good practice. Given the potential breadth of work in this area, it may be useful to set up a sub-group of staff as 'experts'. This group should include a social worker to ensure that carers' assessments are implemented as necessary, and facilitate help with housing, benefits, transport and their own employment as appropriate. Other members of this 'expert' group could gather relevant information for carers; for example, the Rethink guide to practical help for carers; useful websites, local carers' groups (including specific support for minority groups). This information might usefully be kept up to date in a designated area (as described above) where family and friends can feel safe and have some privacy.

The ward team needs to agree the purpose and value of family involvement, and develop an ongoing assessment and support strategy that is implemented by all staff – including receptionist, domestic staff, nursing team and psychiatrist. All need to be positive, supportive and welcoming so that visitors do not feel as though they are 'in the way'. All staff can provide influential role models: through demonstrating trusting, sensitive, clear communication skills, they can help family and friends to realise that although the person might have changed in some way, they are able to make some decisions and take responsibility for their own behaviour. Conversely, staff may learn from family and friends: what the person likes, how he or she relates to people they know well and so on. However, whilst such a general approach is helpful, it is not sufficient: assessment of the wishes and needs of family and friends who normally provide support should become a routine part of every admission.

The involvement of family and friends needs to begin at the point of admission. At initial assessment, the person who is admitted should be asked about living arrangements, the quality of relationships within the family, social contacts and social support. If the family is not present at admission, they must be informed of the admission; wherever family members are involved in supporting the individual, their account and views should be sought, and their needs arising from the relationship must be assessed. Too often it is simply assumed that they are willing and able to continue supporting the person, when further assessment might reveal anxieties about their ability to do so, and doubts about whether they wish to continue in this role. Often individually tailored practical and emotional support will enable them to provide support in a more positive manner, allowing both them and the person admitted to return to a mutually beneficial relationship, and helping both parties to negotiate changed roles as necessary.

The nature of family involvement will vary over time. Initially, the purpose may be to limit disruption and damage to ongoing relationships, supporting the individual and their family as appropriate, providing information to both but giving some respite from relationships that have often been under tremendous pressure. The family may need help to understand the behaviour of the person admitted, how this is managed on the ward and how they can help. They may need 'permission' to visit less frequently, but this is often only possible if they are confident that ward staff are providing secure support, and will contact them if the situation changes. Too often, families report that they have not been given this information; for example, when their relative has absconded and arrives at home when the family thought they were on the ward. Alternatively, families are unhappy with the care provided on the ward; as one mother recounted, 'I didn't like to leave him as he spent all his time lying in bed; they didn't know what to do with him; he only got up when I visited'.

As time goes on, hostility that may be present at admission often decreases, and the purpose of involving the family will be to maintain relationships or provide support and information to improve relationships. Where the person admitted wants their family to be involved, and family members are in agreement, this is often simpler: the family can be involved in planning appropriate support during the admission, and in providing care if they wish. Visiting will be encouraged, with access to a private area for them to meet. Keyworkers will ensure that they speak to family members on a regular basis: answering questions, ensuring that they are aware of progress, treatment, plans, meetings, limitations on leaving the ward, and activities that they can helpfully engage in: taking the person out/home for short periods, on a regular basis. It may be useful to have a message book in the visitors' room for family and friends to record their comments on support provided or, more specifically, they may be encouraged to record their views on progress and treatment.

There are other more specific ways of helping families and friends to support the person admitted to an in-patient unit. 'Psychosocial interventions' have proved helpful for patients in in-patient settings (see Drury et al., 1996): meetings with the individual and those involved in supporting them to discuss the nature of their difficulties and arrive at an understanding about ways of communicating that may be less stressful for all parties. Both families and people with mental health problems want more information on preventing relapse: identifying early signs and devising a clear plan of action for subsequent relapse. These are most effective when family members or close friends work with the individual to arrive at a plan that they all have confidence in. However, it is essential that all parties (services, the patient and nominated supporters) are fully engaged in the process or the responsibility on 'carers' may feel onerous and plans may not be implemented (see Birchwood, 1998).

While a great deal of attention has been paid to the involvement of families in recent years, the maintenance of links with, and support for, friends has been relatively ignored, often leading to the loss of important friendships. On admission, people should be asked about their friendships and offered help to tell their friends that they have been admitted: a person's chances of resuming friendships after admission are jeopardised if they simply 'disappear' from their social networks without explanation. If the person wishes it, friends should be encouraged to visit, staff should be prepared to help the person to explain their problems. It can be difficult for friends to see a person behaving in uncharacteristic and sometimes disturbing ways, and friends need to understand the nature of the person's difficulties if they are to help and support them.

Throughout the admission, efforts must be made to prevent the loss of relationships with family and friends and help the person to resume these relationships when they are able to do so. However, social inclusion involves more than friendships. The things that people do – access to other roles and activities – are equally important.

Roles and activities

The focus of acute care has traditionally been the treatment of symptoms, and relief (asylum) from ordinary activities and responsibilities. However, because of the stigma associated with mental health problems and psychiatric admission, on discharge people face the awkward and sometimes embarrassing task of explaining their absence and trying to resume their ordinary activities and responsibilities. Given the discrimination and stereotypes that surround mental health problems, such efforts are not infrequently unsuccessful. However, if efforts are made to support and increase the understanding of employers, colleges, faith communities, those involved in leisure pursuits and so forth, and support the individual in returning to them, opportunities for re-engagement can be considerably enhanced.

One way of working out how to maintain activities and contacts is to use a weekly diary to record a person's usual routine – before their problems became disabling. This involves spending time with the person discussing the way they spent their week: who they saw when and where, what they did in the evenings, how often they went out, where to. Taking the week on a day-by-day basis provides a structure for this discussion, whilst questions about less frequent but nonetheless important events can also be recorded. This is an important conversation because it confirms that the person is more than just their illness: it goes beyond their problems, and confirms their valued roles and relationships in the community. Many of us do not have buzzing social lives, but we may go to the pub once a week, visit the gym, see siblings once a fortnight or attend church, the library, slimming club. All of these activities count, they give an insight into a person's life outside the ward and are invaluable in planning their support and recovery.

Once significant relationships have been identified, ways of maintaining contact can be planned with the person. There may be a natural wish to hide away from friends and colleagues whilst in hospital – but service users repeatedly emphasise the important role of activities and social contacts in their recovery. Continuing contact with the world outside the mental health system is important in reassuring the person that their life has not stopped with admission: that they can still have a life apart from their mental health difficulties, a role other than that of mental patient. Such continuing contact can be achieved in two ways.

First, given support (some people may want a nurse to be present at first), information as appropriate, and a safe and private place to meet on the ward, friends, colleagues and other social contacts are often pleased to be invited. Second, particularly as the admission progresses, it may be possible for the person to continue some activities while they are in hospital. For example, they may be able to go to church or other religious ceremonies, visit friends, go out for an evening or engage in some sporting activities while they are in hospital. It is not unknown for people to retain some work activity while in hospital, especially when the acute crisis begins to subside. It is often easier for a person to resume some of their activities from the supportive base of an in-patient setting, rather than try to do this with the relatively lower levels of assistance available after discharge. Discharge can be a very difficult time: the *Confidential Enquiry into Homicides and Suicides by Mentally Ill People* (DoH, 1999b) shows that most suicides occur in the week following discharge. If a person is helped to resume their usual activities, and thus gain access to the support and involvement that these entail, then the transition is likely to be easier than returning home alone with nothing to do. Identifying the person's usual activities can also assist in discharge planning and arranging the support that a person may need.

Continued contact during a hospital admission can strengthen relationships and friendships, reduce the stigma of the individual's problems, and ultimately reduce discrimination against mental illness in general. Friends, colleagues and other social contacts are often willing to visit those who have physical problems: they know more or less what to expect and how to behave. If more people were encouraged to visit, psychiatric wards could become less alien places, less removed from the local population.

Many admissions are repeat admissions, and people may have very few friends and an impoverished routine, with all social contacts associated with mental health services. The task then becomes helping people to re-establish new activities and social contacts to regain those that have been lost. An admission can be a good time to help people to begin this process, which might usefully also involve their community care coordinator. First, it is important to establish their interests, wishes and abilities, to generate ideas and discuss opportunities. This requires a knowledge on the part of ward staff about what is available in the local area: education, work and training opportunities; social and leisure facilities; support and self-help groups; religious communities and so forth. The acute admission also offers an opportunity to provide people with support to try out activities before their discharge. Such support may be provided by ward staff, but community staff, friends and relatives, as well as volunteers/befrienders, can also play a role. 'Circles Network', an organisation based in Bristol, provides a model of effective support for developing social support for people without natural contacts. They work with the individual to identify one or two people who are willing to provide specified support, and use these people to generate names of others who could provide additional, quite specific and limited support according to everyone's wishes and needs. These circles of support are very successful because people are usually willing to get involved and help out if responsibility is shared, and demands are delimited.

Given the importance of work and employment in promoting social inclusion, increasing social networks, enhancing quality of life and promoting mental and physical health, particular attention should be paid to issues of employment (or education) on acute admission. First it is important to ascertain whether the person is already in employment, or has some form of work as soon as possible after admission.

If the person is in employment, then, if they wish, plans should be made to maintain this employment. To start off with, it may be necessary to establish whether the person has sent a sickness certificate to their employer. It is more likely that the person will lose their job (whether this be paid or voluntary) or their place on a training/education course if they simply fail to turn up: it is preferable that the employer/ college know that their absence results from ill-health. It is often necessary, with the employer's permission, to liaise with the employer in order to maintain the job: it is often possible to support the employer, dispel some of the myths associated with admission to a psychiatric hospital and help the person to negotiate a return to work. If the person works for a larger firm, then contact with their personnel department or occupational health service can be helpful. Once they understand the position, many employers are keen to retain their employee and willing to make adjustments (like part-time working to start off with or being able to contact a support worker if they have difficulties) to enable the person to return to work. The 1995 Disability Discrimination Act provides some protection against discrimination on the grounds of mental health problems and requires employers to make such 'reasonable adjustments' to enable them to work. Ward staff can play an important role in informing people of their rights and helping to negotiate such adjustments with employers. The Disability Rights Commission can be contacted for advice on these matters.

Sometimes the person may not wish to return to the job or course that they have been doing. In such a situation it may be important to help the person to hand in their notice or inform the college that they are leaving, rather than get sacked. If the person leaves in an orderly fashion then they may be in a better position to apply for other jobs/courses (for example, they are more likely to be able to get a reference from their former tutor/employer).

If the person is not in employment or on a course or does not wish to return to their former position, then employment or training opportunities should be considered during their admission: Standard 5 of the National Service Framework for Mental Health (DoH, 1999a) requires that care plans for people with more serious mental health difficulties include 'action needed for employment, education or training or another occupation'. A vocational assessment should address five main areas (Becker and Drake, 1993).

- Current work goals: client's goals, feasibility of the goals.
- Work background: education, work history – previous jobs, reasons for leaving, satisfactory work experiences, problems at work.

- Current adjustment: physical health, endurance, grooming, interpersonal skills, support network, medication management, symptomatology.
- Work skills: job-seeking skills, job skills, aptitude, interests, motivation, work habits relating to attendance, dependability, stress tolerance.
- Other work-related factors: transportation, family support, substance use, expectations regarding personal, financial and social benefits of working.

It is important to note that such an assessment is not designed to ascertain whether the person is able to work, but to assist in planning the action necessary to enable them to gain and sustain employment and achieve a good match between the job and the person's wishes, skills and problems. Research indicates that the support available and the approaches to work/employment which are adopted are more important in determining vocational success than characteristics of the client (Secker and Membury, 2000).

There are a variety of agencies available in the community to assist people in accessing work or training. These include the disability employment advisers in all employment service JobCentres as well as a variety of other statutory and independent sector services. It is important that staff are aware of such local facilities so that they can assist the person in accessing these. Occupational therapists and vocational services within the Trust are likely to be able to assist in this regard, and local colleges often have special needs advisers who can be of assistance in accessing education courses.

Often service users will be unsure about whether or not to tell employers or colleges about their mental health problems. There are no 'right' answers on this issue, so staff should not attempt to tell people what to do in this regard. However, they can assist people to think about the pros and cons of disclosure in making their own decision. If a person discloses their mental health problems then, given the discrimination that exists, they may be less likely to gain a job in the first place (Manning and White, 1995). However, if they fail to disclose problems that later come to light they may be sacked for failing to do so, they may have difficulty in asking for time off for therapy or doctor's appointments and they cannot avail themselves of the protection from discrimination or 'reasonable adjustments' that they may need to make a success of their work that are available under the Disability Discrimination Act.

Conclusion

Although current priorities and staffing levels in acute settings often mitigate against socially inclusive strategies, it is often possible to make some improvements, and to adjust priorities, within existing resources. It is quite apparent that the strategic development of inclusive strategies in acute settings could improve services for all involved. It is essential that services extend their aims beyond the alleviation of symptoms and go beyond 'psychiatric' measurement (of symptoms, length of stay, professionally devised measures of 'satisfaction with services') in evaluating success, to embrace indicators of social functioning and inclusion. Given the evidence that does exist, careful implementation of inclusive practices – in tandem with whole team training, new means of assessment, different use of space on the ward – appears to have the potential to enhance the outcomes of acute care: to improve the experience and outcomes of acute admissions by maintaining and promoting social relationships, enabling people to maintain or access activities and roles, including work and education, and decrease the mystery and suspicion that surrounds acute admission wards. The available evidence would suggest that if social networks and roles, especially work/employment roles, can be promoted, then the need for acute admissions could be reduced, and it is also likely that a broader socially inclusive perspective would make work on acute wards more rewarding for the staff involved.

In summary, a culture needs to be established in which practitioners think about the ward environment and practices from the perspective of patients, relatives and friends. Would we be happy for one of our relatives or ourselves to be admitted to the facility in which we work? Would we feel comfortable visiting a relative or friend there? We cannot stop our efforts to improve the environment we provide until we can answer 'yes' to both of these questions. Sayce believes that social inclusion should be about providing better access to social and economic opportunities for people with mental health problems, which in turn lead to improvements in status and disability. A range of opportunities for users to access should be available and those who choose to undertake them should be fully supported, including making adjustments where necessary (Sayce, 2000). It is clear that acute care teams have an important part to play in this process, the challenge is to begin the process of change – in attitudes, values, priorities and practice.

References

Appleby, L. (2000) 'A new mental health service: high quality and user-led', *British Journal of Psychiatry*, 177: 290–1.

Barham, P. and Hayward, R. (1995) *Relocating Madness: From the Mental Patient to the Person*. London: Free Association Books.

Bartley, M. (1994) 'Unemployment and ill-health: understanding the relationships', *Journal of Epidemiology and Community Health*, 48: 333–7.

Beale, N. and Nethercott, S. (1985) 'Job-loss and family morbidity: a study of factory closure', *Journal of the Royal College of General Practitioners*, 35: 510–14.

Becker, D.R. and Drake, R.E. (1993) *The Individual Placement and Support Model of Supported Employment.* Concord: New Hampshire–Dartmouth Psychiatric Research Center.

Bennett, D. (1975) 'The value of work in psychiatric rehabilitation', *Social Psychiatry*, 5: 224–30.

Birchwood, M. (1998) 'New directions in the psychosocial approach to psychosis', *Journal of Mental Health*, 7 (2): 111–14.

Brenner, S. and Bartell, R. (1983) 'The psychological impact of unemployment: a structural analysis of cross-sectional data', *Journal of Occupational Psychology*, 56: 129–36.

Burchardt, T. (2000) *Enduring Economic Exclusion: Disabled People, Income and Work.* York: Joseph Rowntree Foundation.

Campbell, P. (2000) 'The role of users of psychiatric services in service development – influence not power', *Psychiatric Bulletin*, 25: 87–8.

Chadwick, P. (1996) *Schizophrenia: The Positive Perspective.* London: Routledge.

Creer, C., Sturt, E. and Wykes, T. (1982) 'The role of relatives', in J.K. Wing (ed.), *Long Term Community Care: Experience in a London Borough.* Psychological Medicine, Monograph Supplement 2, pp. 29–39.

Deegan, P.E. (1993) 'Recovering our sense of value after being labelled mentally ill', *Journal of Psychosocial Nursing and Mental Health Services*, 31 (4): 7–11, 33–4.

Department of Health (1997) *Omnibus Survey of Public Attitudes to Mental Illness.* London: DoH.

Department of Health (1999a) *National Service Framework for Mental Health.* London: DoH.

Department of Health (1999b) *Confidential Enquiry into Homicides and Suicides by Mentally Ill People.* London: DoH.

Department of Health (1999c) *National Carers' Strategy.* London: DoH.

Department of Health (2000a) *NHS Plan.* London: DoH.

Department of Health (2000b) *Making It Happen: A Guide to Delivering Mental Health Promotion.* London: DoH.

Dimsdale, J.E., Klerman, G. and Shershow, J.C. (1979) 'Conflict in treatment goals between patients and staff', *Social Psychiatry*, 14: 1–4.

Drury, V., Birchwood, M. and Cochrane, R. (1996) 'Cognitive therapy and recovery from acute psychosis: a controlled trial. 1: impact on psychotic symptoms', *British Journal of Psychiatry*, 169: 593–601.

Duggan, M., Ford, R., Hill, R., Holmshaw, J., McCulloch, A., Warner, L., Muijen, M., Raftery, J., Strong, S. and Wood, H. (1997) *Pulling Together: The Future Roles and Training of Mental Health Staff.* London: Sainsbury Centre for Mental Health.

Dunn, S. (1999) *Creating Accepting Communities. Report of the Mind Inquiry into Social Exclusion and Mental Health Problems.* London: Mind Publications.

Estroff, S. (1993) 'Community mental health services: extinct, endangered or evolving?' Paper presented at the conference 'Mental Health Practices in the Nineties – Changes and Challenges', Silver Springs, Maryland, USA.

Fadden, G. (1997) 'Implementation of family interventions in routine clinical practice following staff training programmes: a major cause for concern', *Journal of Mental Health*, 6: 599–612.

Fadden, G., Bebbington, P. and Kuipers, E. (1987) 'The burden of care: the impact of functional psychiatric illness on the patient's family', *British Journal of Psychiatry*, 150: 285–92.

Fisher, J. (2003) http://www.rethink.org/news+campaigns/your_voice/lifetime.html

Good Practices in Mental Health (GPMH) (1989) *Treated Well?* London: Camden Mental Health Consortium.

Grove, B. (1999) 'Mental health and employment: shaping a new agenda', *Journal of Mental Health*, 8: 131–40.

Health Advisory Service (HAS) (1999) *Avon and Western Wiltshire Mental Health Trust. Review of Specialist Mental Health Rehabilitation Services.* London: HAS.

Holmes-Eber, P. and Riger, S. (1990) 'Hospitalisation and the composition of patients; social networks', *Schizophrenia Bulletin*, 16 (1): 157.

Institute for Health Care Development (IHCD) (1998) *Core Competencies for Mental Health Workers.* NHS Executive Office North West.

Jahoda, M., Lazersfeld, P. and Zeisl, H. (1933) *Marienthal: The Sociography of an Unemployed Community.* London: Tavistock.

Kuipers, E. (2001) 'Involving service users in the rehabilitation process', *'Rehab' Good Practice Network Newsletter*, 4: 3–5.

Leader, A. and Crosby, K. (1998) *Power Tools.* Brighton: Pavilion.

Leete, E. (1988) 'The role of the consumer movement and people with mental illness'. Presentation at the 12th Mary Switzer Memorial Seminar in Rehabilitation, Washington DC, 15–16 June.

Lewis, G. and Sloggett, A. (1998) 'Suicide, deprivation and unemployment: record linkage study', *British Medical Journal*, 317: 1283–6.

Manning, C. and White, P.D. (1995) 'Attitudes of employers to the mentally ill', *Psychiatric Bulletin*, 19: 541–3.

Mental Health Foundation (2001) *Is Anybody There? A Survey of Friendship and Mental Health.* London: Mental Health Foundation.

Mind (2001) *Environmentally Friendly? Patients' Views of Conditions on Psychiatric Wards.* London: Mind.

Moser, K., Fox, J. and Jones, D. (1987) 'Unemployment and mortality: comparisons of the 1971 and 1981 longitudinal study census samples', *British Medical Journal*, 294: 86–90.

Muijen, M. (1997) Opening paper presented at the Sainsbury Centre Summer School, London.

Newnes, C. (1994) 'Defining mental health', *Nursing Times*, 90: 19, 46.

Perkins, R. (1998) 'An act to follow?', *A Life in the Day*, February, 15–20.

Perkins, R.E. and Repper, J. (1996) *Working Alongside People with Long Term Mental Health Problems.* London: Chapman.

Philippe, A. (1988) 'Suicide and unemployment', *Psychologie Medicale*, 20: 380–2.

Philo, G., Henderson, L. and McLaughlin, G. (1993) *Mass Media Representation of Mental Health/Illness: Report for the Health Education Board for Scotland.* Glasgow: Glasgow University.

Platt, S. and Kreitman, N. (1984) 'Trends in parasuicide among unemployed men in Edinburgh 1968–82', *British Medical Journal*, 289: 1029–32.

Pozner, A., Ng, M., Hammond, J. and Shepherd, G. (1996) *Working It Out.* Brighton: Pavilion.

Read, J. (1996) 'What do we want from mental health services?', in J. Read and J. Reynolds (eds), *Speaking Our Minds.* Milton Keynes: Open University Press.

Read, J. and Baker, S. (1996) *Not Just Sticks and Stones. A Survey of the Stigma, Taboos and Discrimination Experienced by People with Mental Health Problems.* London: Mind.

Reeves, A. (1999) 'Skalligrigg House: the development of a user-run crisis house in Birmingham'. Paper presented at the conference 'Recovery: An Alien Concept?', Chamberlin Hotel, Birmingham.

Repper, J. (2000) 'Translating policy into practice: evaluating a multidisciplinary training in psychosocial interventions for people with serious mental health problems'. Unpublished PhD thesis, University of Manchester.

Rose, D. (2001) *Users' Voices.* London: Sainsbury Centre for Mental Health.

Rowland, L.A. and Perkins, R.E. (1988) 'You can't eat, drink or make love eight hours a day: the value of work in psychiatry', *Health Trends*, 20: 75–9.

Sainsbury Centre for Mental Health (SCMH) (2000) *Acute Problems.* London: SCMH.

Sayce, L. (2000) *From Psychiatric Patient to Citizen: Overcoming Discrimination and Social Exclusion.* London: Macmillan.

Secker, J. and Membury, H. (2000) 'The wicked issues in Wales'. Research Paper for Care Programme to Work Conference, Centre for Mental Health Services Development, London.

Shepherd, G. (1984) *Institutional Care and Rehabilitation.* London: Longman.

Shepherd, G., Murray, A. and Muijen, M. (1995) 'Perspectives on schizophrenia: a survey of user, family care and professional views', *Journal of Mental Health*, 4: 403–22.

Simmons, S. (1994) 'Social networks: their relevance to mental health nursing', *Journal of Advanced Nursing*, 19: 281–9.

Smith, R. (1985) 'Bitterness, shame, emptiness, waste: an introduction to unemployment and health', *British Medical Journal*, 291: 124–8.

Social Exclusion Unit (1999) 'What's it all about?' www.cabinet-office.gov.uk/seu/index/faqs.hmtl (Cabinet Office website).

Standing Nursing and Midwifery Advisory Group (SNMAC) (1999) *Addressing Acute Concerns.* London: DoH.

Stewart, J. (1996) 'Unemployment and health. 1: the impact on clients in rehabilitation and therapy', *British Journal of Therapy and Rehabilitation*, 3: 360.

Wallcraft, J. (1994) 'Empowering empowerment: professionals and self-advocacy projects', *Mental Health Nursing*, 14 (2): 6–9.

Warner, R. (1994) *Recovery from Schizophrenia: Psychiatry and Political Economy*, 2nd edn. London: Routledge.

Warr, P. (1987) *Work, Unemployment and Mental Health.* Oxford: Oxford University Press.

Wilson, S. and Walker, G. (1993) 'Unemployment and health: a review', *Public Health*, 107: 153–62.

Winefield, H. and Burnett, P. (1996) 'Barriers to alliance between family and professional care-givers in chronic schizophrenia', *Journal of Mental Health*, 5: 223–32.

Wing, J.K. and Morris, B. (1981) 'Clinical basis of rehabilitation', in J. Wing (ed.), *Handbook of Psychiatric Rehabilitation Practice.* Oxford: Oxford University Press.

FOUR

Strategies for surviving acute care

Alison Faulkner

Introduction

Anyone who has been admitted to an acute in-patient ward in recent years would be forgiven for coming to the conclusion that mental health care is in a serious crisis. Many of our inner city in-patient wards have become merely places of containment and medication. Acute wards have lost their role and focus within the mental health system; they are fought over by the various stakeholders, all of whom have rather different agendas: the public and the media, who are primarily concerned about public safety, patients/ service users who want or need care and treatment in a crisis, and nursing staff and psychiatrists who may believe themselves to have a role in all of these but may be confused as to what their primary focus should be.

The focus of this chapter is the service user or patient within the acute mental health care environment. Whilst much of what I have to say may be critical of existing services, I hope to be able to pinpoint elements of good practice and principles of good and respectful care. I believe that acute mental health care represents a major challenge for the 21st century, and one that we must not fail to address. The mental health nurse has a major role in this; as the staff member with the most (potential) contact with the patient in care, the nurse has the opportunity to effect change at the most fundamental point within the system.

Experiences of acute care

> The proof of the pudding is in the eating, and not from statistics in a textbook or dis-
> charge notes. I regret the day I ever discovered the system. (Lloyd-Jones, 2001: 7)

It is worthwhile first re-visiting the nature of the experience. I make no apology for doing this, despite the critical nature of this review, because it is absolutely vital that we remember what it feels like to be at the receiving end of acute mental health care. Many accounts have been written about the experience of being admitted to an acute psychiatric ward (e.g., Faulkner, 1998; Rose, 2000; Lloyd-Jones, 2001). They make difficult reading, not least because the loss of status and identity, the distress and discrimination associated with mental ill-health, is often compounded by the attitudes and experiences encountered in hospital – a time when what is needed is care and treatment, and assistance in returning home. Without exception, these writers report not being listened to, treatment that sometimes amounts to punishment, coercion and fear, boredom and a lack of information about what is going on in relation to their care and treatment.

In my own experience, long days of watching television and waiting for medication, visiting times or meal times, were underpinned by a total lack of engagement by nursing staff. When I was congratulated by one nurse on dealing with things by myself, I could only wonder at how I had managed to get the whole system so wrong! I was far too terrified to approach anyone for help or to talk to on the ward: nurses were busy, they stayed in the office or watched television and never offered the space or opportunity to talk. All that my fellow patients and I could do in extremity was to express this need for human contact in terms of distress, anger or self-harm.

On the same subject, Hutchison (2000a) states that the reason nurses do not engage users in conversation is often explained by a belief that people should take personal responsibility and ask for help. This, however, fails to recognise how difficult and demeaning it can be for users to approach a group of nurses and ask to speak to someone; a situation exacerbated when often the response is that they will have to wait until the nurse can find the time.

Harsh and/or threatening treatment of patients by nurses can be observed on any short admission. In one month on the ward, I saw two or three patients threatened with the Mental Health Act 1983 for what appeared to be relatively minor 'offences' (such as leaving the ward five minutes early for lunch), and two male patients taunted by a nurse calling them 'poofs':

> some patients, for no other reason than a raised voice, were roughly handled – pinned down by four male staff, given an injection and sent to the infamous seclusion room. (Lloyd-Jones, 2001: 7)

I was myself once threatened with the seclusion room for smashing a cup and saucer; no account was taken of the fact that at the time I had been very distressed by a male patient's unwelcome approaches. Similarly, people who self-harm whilst in hospital are often punished for doing so, rather than treated with some care and an attempt at understanding.

Some of the more frightening aspects of being an in-patient may not be universally experienced. However, the more pervasive and difficult-to-change aspects are also often the simplest or most basic aspects of people caring for people, and do not require enormous resources to change. For example, Hutchison (2000b) advocates treating people with 'dignity and respect'. This principle is so fundamental that it is almost worth a chapter on its own. Many aspects of the care environment and care delivery already mentioned – such as poor hygiene and basic amenities, lack of safety and poor staff attitudes – diminish self-respect on a day-to-day basis. The message is strong: you are not important whilst you are in hospital. You are simply one of many and will get no individual attention or treatment to enable you to feel cared for.

Research

There is considerable evidence now to support the many anecdotal accounts of poor and unsafe care on in-patient acute wards. The Sainsbury Centre for Mental Health (1998) reported on the quality of care in acute psychiatric wards. In their in-depth study of nine wards, they interviewed 112 patients about their care and the environment on the wards. They found, amongst other things, that:

- in-patient care was unpopular amongst patients;
- wards lacked basic amenities; e.g., no separate bedrooms, no lockers, no quiet areas;
- many patients felt unsafe;
- women were particularly dissatisfied: concern about privacy, cleanliness and personal safety were expressed.

Our own research at the Mental Health Foundation (Faulkner, 1997; Faulkner and Layzell, 2000) supports the demand for more person-centred care. Over and over again, people expressed the wish for 'someone to talk to' or human contact and support during times of crisis and distress. In the survey reported in *Knowing Our Own Minds* (Faulkner, 1997), the majority of people when asked the question 'What do you feel you need when in distress?', responded that they wanted someone to talk to and/or support from other people. For some, this was a general expression of need, whilst for others it concerned a specific person or people.

More recently, Mind carried out a survey on conditions in psychiatric units (Hunter, 2000). Compiled from the accounts of 340 people with recent experience of hospital admission, it describes the experience as untherapeutic, depressing and frequently unsafe. Fifty-seven per cent of patients said they did not get enough time with staff, with many reporting that contact with staff amounted to between only 5 and 15 minutes a day. Mind recommends 'more genuine and meaningful consultation with users of mental health services' as a means of achieving a service truly responsive to the needs of its users.

Possible explanations

There are, I think, a number of reasons for the distressing circumstances described above, which I have outlined elsewhere (Faulkner, 1998).

Resources. Insufficient or inappropriately allocated resources – whether financial or human – are often given as the basis for a service maintaining the status quo (Audit Commission, 1994).

Adherence to the medical model. Whilst mental health problems remain the domain of the medical profession, solutions or treatments will be limited accordingly – often to the use of medication. However, evidence suggests that what people want in a mental health crisis is someone to talk to, human contact and support (Rogers et al., 1992; Faulkner, 1997). This is not what acute services are geared up to provide. In general, changes to a service which do not fit with the medical model – as is often the case with the alternatives proposed by service users – are not acceptable or are more difficult to achieve than those that do. It is for this reason that service users are increasingly looking to develop their own alternatives outside of the statutory services (Lindow, 1994).

One of the more serious implications of the medical model is the invalidation of the individual and his/her views. This can often lead to treatment and care delivery that does not fully include or involve the patient or service user, on apparently valid grounds. Yet, people continue to be whole human beings throughout periods of distress, and can be consulted about their views and involved in their treatment.

The political context. It is an unfortunate reality that mental health services have multiple clients: service users, carers, professionals and 'society' at large. At present the political context appears to be supporting society's agenda, as evidenced by the response to media images of dangerousness and the risks of community care, and the Mental Health Act White Paper. The danger of this focus is that acute services may become simply the tool of social control with the result that the interface between mental health professional and service user becomes more conflicting than it is at present.

The culture or institutionalisation of a service can also serve to block change whether in a local specific service, such as a ward or day centre, or in relation to the broader environment. Either way, it is hard for individuals to change or to fight against a dominant culture if it is based on the power of maintaining the status quo. A new nurse on the ward fresh out of radical nurse training, might simply fit in with the general approach taken, rather than risk standing out or being ostracised by his or her colleagues.

A fear of engaging with people as individuals is an issue that seems paramount but also represents a question to which I do not know the answer. Does discrimination influence the staff working in mental health services as much as the service users and the public in general – and create a greater barrier between staff and clients – a greater 'them and us' culture in which the meaning of people's lives becomes denied? Certainly it is my experience that the *meaning* of mental distress is more the preserve of fellow service users and survivors, than it is of the mental health service professionals. It is amongst ourselves that we talk honestly and openly about what we do and feel, and why we think that might be. When faced with a doctor or a nurse, it is often the case that we are afraid of their possible response and so censor ourselves.

Staff morale is an issue that pervades much of this discussion. Coming back to the beginning of the chapter, and the focus on people's experiences, my concern is that staff morale is being affected by an increasingly custodial approach to care which has developed out of the negative images of risk and dangerousness. This may well contrast with a more therapeutic approach for which they might have expected to go into the profession in the first place. Stigma, or discrimination as it is more realistically experienced by people, may be affecting staff within mental health services almost as much as it is affecting the person on the street (Dodd, 1998), who is forming an impression of mental illness as a cause only of aggression and dangerous behaviour, not a cause for understanding, care or for treatment. The result may well be deterioration of relationships between nurses and patients, both of whom are on the immediate frontline of this battle for a service.

User involvement

The term 'user involvement' tends to be used with some carelessness these days, and it can mean very different things to different people. With all of the policy exhortations to involve consumers, you would be forgiven for thinking it was all pretty much solved, or at least widely accepted. The Patient's Charter (DoH, 1992) and the National Service Framework for Mental Health (DoH, 1999) placed mental health service users in a more central position within community care policy. However, user involvement can certainly be approached in a superficial or tokenistic manner by some service providers, rather than becoming a meaningful or genuine process.

It is useful in this context to think about user involvement at two different levels: the individual and the service levels. The distinction is an important one, as they can serve quite different purposes even if they share significant agendas.

User involvement at the individual level

At the individual level, it is important that users feel heard and listened to, that services and staff are responding to the needs we express, and that our treatment whilst in hospital has some meaning to us as individuals. Users want to be consulted and involved in decisions about our treatment and care.

Over the last two decades there have been initiatives and policy directives that attempt to re-state the role of consumer rather than as passive recipient, patient or service user. Mental health service consumers are supposed to be involved in the drawing up of care plans and actively participate in the Care Programme Approach (CPA) (DoH, 1991) review process. However, a recent report by the User Focused Monitoring team at the Sainsbury Centre for Mental Health (Rose, 2001) shows that people are rarely involved in care planning – in fact, the majority of users in one area did not know that they had a care plan. Similarly, the research found a total lack of involvement in the CPA review process. Rose concludes that the demands of the user movement and of policy makers are not being heard when it comes to the day-to-day organisation and delivery of services.

Information is one of the keys to involvement. The need for information – on a range of mental health, community care and life-related issues – is of paramount importance when planning care provision. A study carried out jointly by the Mental Health Foundation and the National Association of Citizens' Advice Bureaux (Bird and Majumdar, 1998) found that, for service users, there was often an unmet need for information and advice. Without such information, users cannot know what they are letting themselves in for when admitted to hospital, nor what choices may be available. Information, after all, is power.

Second, it seems to me that there is a need to make the benefits of user involvement more explicit to staff. An interesting finding from the report is that users who were involved in the care planning process were more likely to be satisfied with the services they received. Whilst Rose points out that this cannot necessarily be seen as 'cause and effect', it is nevertheless an interesting indicator of the value of involvement.

Advocacy, crisis cards, advance directives

The experiences reported above, especially if repeated over years of contact with services, erode self-esteem and reduce the sense of individual power. How, then, can some degree of power be reinstated?

One approach towards maximising user involvement at the individual level is the use of advocacy. Advocacy – stated simply – is the opportunity to have someone alongside you who will voice your concerns for you if you wish them to. Many people (and I count myself among them) may be articulate for most of the time, but in the face of a ward round consisting of a number of professionals, can be reduced to the silence of stone. Peter Campbell (2001) supports the value of independent advocacy: the ability to make a personal choice of advocate, regardless of their training or qualifications, because it is the personal alliance that matters. He questions whether advocacy 'works', in the sense of securing better results, but believes that having someone on your side throughout your experiences is worth fighting for.

Crisis cards, on the other hand, may have a practical use that will enable their value to be appreciated by service providers and service users alike. They were originally conceived of as advocacy tools, to enable people to contact someone on behalf of the card carrier, who would offer support in a crisis. In some places where crisis cards have been implemented, their use has become somewhat more elaborate and often service-focused – with named keyworker, sometimes services, and even information about medication.

These additions may not detract from their original intention (to ensure that the person experiencing a mental health crisis receives the help they want) so long as they are drawn up with the full consent and involvement of the card carrier. Difficulties may emerge in situations where the card becomes more complex and more negotiation with mental health workers is required.

Which brings us to advance directives. An advance directive (also known as a 'living will') allows someone to make decisions before they become ill, about their future treatment. These decisions cannot be ignored unless:

- the advance directive does not apply to the particular situation which arises;
- the advance directive is not clear;
- or if the Mental Health Act is used to override a person's intentions regarding treatment.

Advance directives are designed to establish – and, essentially, communicate to others – a person's preferences for treatment should they become incompetent to express these in the future to treatment providers. The principle behind an advance directive is to enhance an individual's ability to exert a measure of control or choice over times in their life when they are in extreme distress, or lose the ability to express themselves or their treatment preferences. The advance directive has a particular value in mental health, where an individual's competence is likely to fluctuate.

Only advance refusals of treatment have any existing legal status (although even these may be overruled under the Mental Health Act 1983 if they concern treatment for 'mental disorder'). So, although advance preferences may not be followed by medical practitioners if they contradict clinical advice, advance statements may take the approach of specifying preferences (e.g., one drug against another), or simple refusals of a particular type of treatment, as well as naming a personal contact or advocate. In this way, advance statements may well ameliorate a crisis situation, avoid a section or enable the individual to exercise some control over a potentially uncontrollable situation.

User involvement at the service level

It is not easy to become 'involved' in an acute in-patient service: by its very nature, it is unlikely to be a service that is encouraging long-term admission or involvement from its users. However, there are some significant ways in which service users can be consulted about or involved in the way in which the service is delivered.

Hutchison (2000b) suggests that service users should be involved in:

- the planning of their own support;
- the design and running of statutory and independent services;
- the recruitment of staff;
- the training of mental health professionals;
- monitoring the effectiveness of services;
- researching and evaluating services;
- the establishment of user-run or user-led services.

This gives us rather a lot to do, and presents a number of challenges! However, Hutchison's basic premise is that there is a need for a fundamental shift in the balance of power if users are to regain some control over their lives. Nowhere is this more true, I would argue, than in the acute setting, where control is most likely to be in the hands of the professionals, whether one is detained under the Mental Health Act or not.

Meaningful user involvement at the local service level can mean attending appropriately to weekly ward meetings: taking notes of comments and complaints, and responding to them. My experience of one ward meeting was that the nurse in charge simply responded 'there's nothing I can do about that' to nearly all of the comments made by patients, most of which concerned basic amenities and hygiene. There is no point in holding ward meetings for the apparent benefit of patients if there can be no positive outcomes for patients. They can be used positively to monitor change and service response over time.

Whilst it has become fairly commonplace for services to invite service users onto planning committees or forums, it is rare for this to be thought through and enacted in a meaningful way such that the service users can feel like equal members or partners in the process. Often this is because the services in question are fulfilling a directive from above that states a need for there to be 'user involvement' without any real understanding of, or commitment to, that concept. There are a few simple guidelines for user involvement to be more than just tokenism:

- ensure that there is more than one service user on a committee;
- pay people for their time and expenses, unless they are being paid from another source like the professionals on that committee;
- be clear and honest about the limits of involvement and influence;
- if necessary, give people training in the workings of committees;
- ensure all information and papers are written in clear, accessible language and any jargon is fully explained;
- provide people with access to support to attend, if required.

Finally, for user involvement at this level to be meaningful, it has to engage more service users than the two or three who are attending a meeting. Ideally, those service users will be part of a wider group – perhaps a local user group – and will be able to feed in the views of other local service users as well as feed back to them about the workings and decisions of the committee. This therefore has implications for the support of local user groups. A genuine commitment to greater service user involvement in all aspects of service design and delivery has to be demonstrated through the encouragement and material support of user self-organisations. Care should also be taken to ensure that such groups maintain their autonomy of thought and are not incorporated into 'management' (Barnes et al., 1999). Of course, it should not be assumed that all service users or user groups wish to be 'involved' in their local services; many wish to focus their energies on developing alternative supports and services within and for the group.

Back to basics ...

User involvement is important and indeed vital for significant change to take place in the understanding and delivery of acute in-patient care.

However, there are some fundamental issues that can happen now, and need no significant resources to implement. People – who become patients or service users – are people and need to be treated as such. The experience of hospital admission can be improved by examining current practice through a few simple exercises. The video and training package *This Could be You*, produced by the Royal Edinburgh Hospital Patients' Council (2000) represents an excellent starting point. The video takes the viewer(s) through three sections.

1. How would you feel if this was you?
2. How can you exercise control in a sensitive and empowering way?
3. Are you institutionalised?

This encourages trainees to see hospital admission from the patient's perspective. What is it like to be admitted to hospital, not knowing the rules or routines, and not knowing what to expect? Working in the same hospital environment for many years is likely to make it hard for nurses to imagine what it is like to be admitted for the first time. It is easy to take the environment and regular practices for granted and to assume that people will know what to expect; the truth is that many people are quite shocked and bewildered by the experience and need help and support to adjust to it.

Returning to the results of the Mental Health Foundation's *Strategies for Living* research, the things that people valued through their strategies and supports reflected finding themselves valued as human beings. People talk about such concepts as feeling accepted by others and finding self-acceptance, the importance of emotional support, finding ways of sharing experiences and sharing an essential aspect of their identity, finding meaning and purpose and a reason for living. Some also talked about taking control over their lives, and the importance of finding security, safety and peace. Not all of these are sought or expected within an acute setting, but it is easy to see how the latter might fail people in some of these areas.

Barker (2000) talks about the 'tidal model' of nursing care, which aims to put the needs of the individual service user at the centre. Whilst the sailing analogy is something of an anathema to me, the three dimensions of caring described seem to hold a great deal of potential for improving patient care.

- In the 'world' dimension, the nurse focuses on the person's need to be understood. This includes a need to have the personal experience of distress, illness or trauma, validated by others.
- In the 'self' dimension, the nurse focuses on the person's need for emotional and physical security.

- In the 'others' dimension, the care plan considers the kind of support that might be provided by other disciplines or agencies, in order to resolve immediate problems or lead an ordinary life.

These 'dimensions' have implications for direct care. For example, the 'world' dimension leads to an holistic nursing assessment which enables documentation of what is significant and meaningful to the person at the present time, and identifies what needs to happen next. The assessment and care plan are written in the person's own words, a simple means of reducing the disempowerment inherent in a clinical and medical-based system.

I do not believe that there is a single right approach to nursing in the acute setting – only the need to improve or change the current situation. It is simply not acceptable in the 21st century for people to have this kind of experience:

> It is quite possible, even common, for a close-observations nurse to have no interaction whatever with the patient during an eight-hour shift. … This lack of communication is harmful in itself. It makes you feel controlled without being helped, and scrutinised like a specimen rather than a human being. (Rose, 2000: 8)

References

Audit Commission (1994) *Finding a Place*. London: HMSO.

Barker, P. (2000) 'Turning the tide', *Openmind*, 106: 10–11.

Barnes, M., Harrison, S., Mort, M., and Shardlow, P. (1999) *Unequal Partners: User Groups and Community Care*. Bristol: Policy Press.

Bird, L. and Majumdar, A. (1998) *MHF Briefing Paper No. 14: CAB Services for People with Mental Health Problems: Paper for Mental Health Services, Purchasers and Commissioners*. London: Mental Health Foundation.

Campbell, P. (2001) *Something Inside So Strong*. London: Mental Health Foundation.

Department of Health (1991) *The Care Programme Approach*. London: HMSO.

Department of Health (1992) *The Patient's Charter*. London: HMSO.

Department of Health (1999) *National Service Framework for Mental Health*. London: The Stationery Office.

Dodd, T. (1998) 'The social construction of the mental health service user', *Mental Health Practice*, 8: 6.

Faulkner, A. (1997) *Knowing Our Own Minds*. London: Mental Health Foundation.

Faulkner, A. (1998) 'Experts by experience', *Mental Health Nursing*, 18 (4): 6–8.

Faulkner, A. and Layzell, S. (2000) *Strategies for Living: A Report of User-Led Research into People's Strategies for Living with Mental Distress*. London: Mental Health Foundation.

Hunter, M. (2000) 'Service needs user input', *Community Care*, 16–22 November, p. 12.

Hutchison, M. (2000a) *Looking to the Future*. London: Mental Health Foundation.

Hutchison, M. (2000b) 'Issues around empowerment', in T. Basset (ed.), *Looking to the Future: Key Issues for Contemporary Mental Health Services*. Brighton: Pavilion/ Mental Health Foundation.

Lindow, V. (1994) *Self-help Alternatives to Mental Health Services*. London: Mind.

Lloyd-Jones, V. (2001) 'No toothpaste', *Openmind*, 107: 7.

Rogers, A., Pilgrim, D. and Lacey, R. (1992) *Experiencing Psychiatry: Users' Views of Services*. London: Mind.

Rose, D. (2000) 'A year of care', *Openmind*, 106: 8.

Rose, D. (2001) *Users' Voices: The Perspectives of Mental Health Service Users on Community and Hospital Care*. London: Sainsbury Centre for Mental Health.

Royal Edinburgh Hospital Patients' Council (2000) *This Could Be You: A Service User's Training Guide for Clinical and Other Staff Working in Hospital with People with Mental Health Problems*. Brighton: Pavilion.

Sainsbury Centre for Mental Health (1998) *Acute Problems: A Survey of the Quality of Care in Acute Psychiatric Wards*. London: Sainsbury Centre for Mental Health.

FIVE

Case management: perspectives of the UK and US systems

Martin Ward and Gail W. Stuart

Introduction

Health care organisations around the world are seeing increased demand for services, escalating costs, limited resources and difficulty with access to care for health care consumers. Case management has been seen as one strategy that could positively impact health care by serving as a gate-keeper and ensuring quality, as well as cost-effective, care. Case management was not developed solely for mental illness and indeed some of its major successes have arisen as a consequence of combining it with the nursing process and primary nursing in the provision of care for a variety of general medical specialties in hospital settings. As will be seen in this chapter, this is not the way it has developed within mental health. Case management is defined by the Case Management Society of America (1995: 8) as a

> collaborative process that assesses, plans, implements, coordinates, monitors, and evaluates the options and services required to meet an individual's health needs, using communication and available resources to promote quality, cost-effective outcomes.

Within the mental health setting, case management is an umbrella term used to describe a variety of approaches for providing community support for those people suffering from severe and persistent mental illness. It was first developed within the United States in the late 1970s (Stein et al., 1975; Stein and Test, 1980), not as a therapeutic process, but more as a way of coordinating agencies to meet the needs of this target group. In the United Kingdom, it has been conceived as a method of linking discharge packages with long-term and intensive community support. As such, it constitutes the underlying structure for assertive outreach (Andrews and Teesson, 1994).

Although case management in mental health delivery systems has been adopted in many countries worldwide and despite claims for its effectiveness (Rubin, 1992), there remain concerns about its efficacy (Marshall et al., 1997), its philosophical and organisational structures (Rothman, 1992), its role as either a therapeutic tool or a brokerage system for coordinating packages of care (Ryan et al., 1991; Bergen, 1994), and even its typology (Thornicroft, 1991). Thus many clinical and research questions remain to be addressed in the implementation and evaluation of case management programmes in psychiatric care.

A synthesis of the available literature and research suggests that the following are commonly accepted components of effective case management.

- A comprehensive assessment of the individual's needs.
- Development of a care plan or package of care to meet those needs.
- Ensuring that the individual has access to or receives the care that is needed; this may involve assertive outreach work on the part of the case manager.
- Monitoring the quality of care provided.
- Monitoring ongoing, long-term support and contact with the individual.

The need for case management in mental health

Many problems exist related to the provision of services to the severely mentally ill, including:

- ignorance of how to obtain and maintain support services;
- inability to perform self-care activities;
- problems in obtaining and remaining in housing;
- difficulty coping with daily stressors and financing daily needs;
- lack of concordance with treatment plans and medication regimen;
- problems obtaining and receiving medical care.

Vigorous clinical management approaches are needed to coordinate care in ways that are responsive to the needs of the severely mentally ill across numerous and complex areas, while decreasing the problem of service fragmentation and containing costs. Case management in mental health was developed to coordinate the housing, financial support, psychiatric treatment and primary health care needs for those clients lacking the skills and resources to accomplish these goals for themselves.

Clearly, the provision of case management services for people with severe and persistent mental health problems is both costly and time-consuming if it is to be successful. However, such a statement cannot be considered lightly because one needs to establish what outcomes clients and care providers expect, what resources are already available within existing provisions and just what is meant by 'successful'? People do not always 'recover' from mental illness in the same way that they do from physical illnesses.

From a case management perspective there are distinct similarities between those with mental health problems and those suffering the physical consequences of serious accidents or chronic illnesses. In both cases there may be no ability for independent living without outside help, no expectation of total recovery or returning to one's pre-illness life, and no relief from a growing dependency on specially trained skilled help to ensure the safety of the vulnerable individual. The main differences may only be in the perception of others as to the necessity for such help, and the financial determination of the health care system to support such people over time. A person suffering the effects of physical illness is easily identifiable as requiring such help. A person suffering a loss of social skills and debilitated by intrusive thoughts and bizarre beliefs is most often not as easily recognised or supported.

Financial resources are finite and some degree of prioritisation has to be undertaken to ensure that the needs of the majority are met within limited health care budgets. This focus on generalised health care holds the key to understanding some of the problems associated with mental health case management. In the case of chronic physical illness the situation is both obvious and the alternatives, in terms of cost of in-patient care or to the person's quality of life, make the provision of individualised, complex and personalised community care viable. The need is clear, but so too is the demand from society that it should be met appropriately. This combination of available and cost-effective social and health care options and pressure influenced by social conscience is a powerful bargaining tool for the individual requiring such help. Unfortunately, for a variety of reasons the same tool is not ordinarily available to those suffering from the effects of severe mental illness.

Although mental illness may affect as many as one in six people within Western societies, health budget allocations seldom reflect this statistic. Despite official rhetoric to the opposite, mental health care across countries is often a poor relation to that for physical health. Deprived of the funds that would enable it to offer a diversity of care options, it has consistently had to target blanket care options to deal with the needs of the majority of its service users. The availability of financial resources for sophisticated long-term care is therefore dependent upon very careful budgetary management and recognition on the part of planners that money would be well spent on such activities.

There is a significant body of longitudinal research showing that patients suffering from enduring mental health problems, when eventually discharged from in-patient care, not only improve, but, if given the right kind of support, become well established within society. For example, Leff and Trieman (2000), reporting on aspects of the five-year TAPS project, showed that of the 670 discharged patients included in the survey, most gained domestic and community living skills, acquired friends and confidants, and were living in freer conditions with the majority wanting to remain in the current homes.

The role of nursing in case management

The concept of case management appears to be universal to the delivery of health care. The term appears in social work, nursing, health economics and political reform literature. The role of the case manager has emerged from these disciplines as a proposed panacea for clients, providers and payers in an attempt to optimise health and conserve resources. Many goals have been suggested for case management. These include maximising the client's self-care capacities, promoting the more efficient use of resources, and stimulating the creation of new services. Other goals include providing quality care across a continuum, decreasing the fragmentation of care across settings, enhancing the client's quality of life and cost containment. Case management has also been suggested as a way of fostering consumer participation in decision-making related to health and advocacy in systems for consumer outcomes (ANA, 1991).

Some believe that case management is something that nurses have always done making the point that public health nurses have been case managing for years. Others suggest that nurses as case managers are the direct result of the managed care movement in America (Wrinn, 1998). Regardless, it is clear that nurses are uniquely prepared to serve as case managers within health care settings (Glettler and Leen, 1996). Coordinating care and clinical health skills are integral to the professional practice of nursing. So too, the caring philosophy of nursing is congruent with the goals of case management. Nurses focus on interactive, caring relationships which optimise client-directed goals for health and well-being. It has also been noted that the need for case managers to possess expertise in clinical practice has in part been responsible for the shift in case management providers from predominantly social workers to nursing professionals (Mullahy, 1998).

In fact there is a rich literature describing: the roles of nurses as case managers in general medical health care settings; core components of successful nurse case management programmes; and barriers to the development and success of such programmes (Glettler and Leen, 1996; Doyle, 2001). There is a somewhat smaller literature focusing on: the role of psychiatric nurses as case managers for the seriously mentally ill (Atkinson, 1996; Firn, 1997); nurses case managing those persons with diagnoses other than schizophrenia (Nehls, 2001); and case management in consultation/liaison services (Chase et al., 2000). Nonetheless, nurses' involvement in case management programmes in mental health delivery systems around the world continues to be examined and valued (Burns et al., 2001).

Within mental health, case managers generally work within a community setting. To distinguish them from traditional community psychiatric staff it is necessary to explore some of the practical considerations that they face.

1. They act as the primary contact between care services and the patient. This often begins by visiting the patient whilst still an in-patient, developing a working relationship with them and establishing a partnership. This partnership, or contract, is different from an ordinary clinical role in that the case manager is not responsible for administering medication, though of course will observe its impact and work with the patient to ensure that they maintain their treatment regimes. Also, a case manager will not normally take responsibility for invoking formal re-hospitalisation thus taking the role of a professional friend rather than a health care agent. Nothing is technically speaking outside of this relationship if it supports and protects the patient.

2. The patient may be accompanied by the case manager on discharge and if not will certainly meet with them on the day of discharge. As the case manager has a much smaller caseload than a traditional community nurse, on average about 15 patients, more time will be spent with each of those patients. Following discharge this may be as much as two or three times a day or an equivalent in time.

3. The patient, not the treatment regimes, will determine the contract between the two. Time will initially be spent getting to know each other, building up mutual trust and exploring what needs to be done as a priority. The case manager will also work with the patient's relatives and primary carers if this is appropriate, though it has to be agreed with the patient if this is to be the case.

4. Irrespective of the case manager's background, be it social or health care and in some cases an ex-patient themselves, much of their work will be in a supportive role. Helping with the decorating may be just as much a priority for a patient as claiming their social security benefits and both of these will be the active realms of the case manager.

5. Meetings between the two, though pre-arranged, are informal and generally occur in the patient's home. However, they are just as likely to be in a café, a park or a place of the patient's choosing. The whole purpose of case management is to centre on the needs of the patient,

and this cannot be done if they are expected to always meet with the case manager on his/her home soil; i.e., a clinic or health facility.

6. The case manager will leave his/her contact details with the patient and is effectively on call for them 24 hours a day, 7 days a week.

7. As time progresses the amount of contact between case manager and patient will decrease, by mutual agreement. However, case managers seldom discharge patients from their caseload, even if they have to be re-admitted to in-patient care. The main reasons for absolute case management discharge are that the two have irreconcilable differences and a new case manager has to be appointed, that the patient becomes self-supporting and can be transferred to lower levels of supervision from other community workers, or the patient dies. Of course, financial pressures and resource disposition can mean that not enough case managers are available, and under these extreme circumstances patients may have to be transferred to other agencies even though in theory they ought to remain with the case manager.

8. If a patient has to be re-admitted to an in-patient facility, often the case manager will accompany them, visit them whilst admitted and work with the patient to plan for their discharge.

9. The case manager reports back to the multidisciplinary team about patient progress and to receive case supervision. Case management is very time- and resource-consuming. For the case manager, often working so autonomously, it can also cause great stress and 'burn-out'. Supervision, the need to feel part of a working team and sensitive line-management are essential ingredients for the successful ongoing support of active case managers (Ward et al., 1999).

Inevitably the nurse's professional background will influence the way they establish the relationship with the patient. And, whilst their interactions with them will hopefully be of therapeutic value, the nurse, as a case manager, is not there to provide therapy as such. For example, a patient may require a complex package of care that includes medication, counselling, some form of occupational therapy and social training. The case manager will monitor the effects of medication, encourage the patient to maintain contact with those nurses who give that medication and, if necessary, report back to those nurses adverse effects and non-concordance with the treatment regime. He/she will not give the medication themselves.

Similarly, they will ensure that the patient gets to the counselling session, to the occupational therapy session or to see any other specialist therapist identified within the care package and, again, monitor the effects of this work. Discussing these things with the patient, reinforcing the work of the therapists and gauging the patient's response to them represent the case manager's role within the therapy process.

Social training may be the only exception to this rule. Again, where specialist help is required (i.e., in gaining benefits, housing and perhaps employment) the case manager will put the patient in contact with the expert in this area, often accompanying them to meetings and appointments. They will help them complete forms and discuss the options open to them but they will not actually do the work of these agencies. They may, however, work within the social training programme to develop the patient's social skills, help them with domestic activities such as shopping, home decorating or gardening, and work to create a social environment by enabling the patient to meet with friends and relatives. The role here is a supportive one but hopefully it is also one where the patient gradually learns to do these things for him/herself. The case manager is just as likely to be enjoying an afternoon with the patient discussing the colour of the wallpaper as he/she is being called out at 3 a.m. responding to that same patient's call for help in a personal or clinical crisis.

Case management in the United States

In the United States, case management has been a commonly used model of service delivery in public-sector mental health settings for almost three decades (Sabin, 1998). Most recently, private-sector behavioural health companies have also adopted it. It was originally conceived as a means of providing comprehensive and continuous care to newly deinstitutionalised persons with severe mental illness (Bachrach, 1981). Over time, however, the meaning of case management has become more ambiguous and complex. Definitions, goals and models of case management now vary widely depending on the organisational philosophy and structure of the mental health delivery system.

'Case management' in the US is often an ambiguous term that can refer to radically different activities ranging from expansive efforts to increase access to care to restrictive efforts to reduce costs through applications of 'medical necessity'. Such efforts to increase access to care are primarily associated with the public sector, while restrictive efforts are associated with the private sector. The most successful programme would be one that combines public-sector receptivity and asylum with driven private-sector efficiency (Sledge et al., 1995).

Case management has been defined in various ways. Solomon (1992), for example, distinguished four types of case management: assertive community treatment, strengths case management, rehabilitation, and generalist case management. Mueser and colleagues (1998) described six models: broker case management, clinical case management, strengths case management, rehabilitation case management, assertive community treatment,

Table 5.1 Components and interventions of clinical case management

Component	Intervention
Initial phase	Engagement Assessment Planning
Environmental interventions	Linkages with community resources Consultation with families and caregivers Maintenance and expansion of social networks Collaboration with physicians and hospitals Advocacy
Patient interventions	Individual psychotherapy Training in independent living skills Psychoeducation
Patient–environment interventions	Crisis intervention Monitoring

Source: B. Greco and N. Worley (2001) 'Community psychiatric nursing care', in G. Stuart and M. Laraia (eds), *Principles and Practice of Psychiatric Nursing*. St Louis, MO: Mosby. pp. 728–43.

and intensive case management. Perhaps the most commonly used conceptualisation of case management distinguishes between *case management* and *assertive community treatment*.

Case management services are aimed at linking the service system to the consumer and coordinating the service components so that he or she can achieve successful community living. It includes problem solving to provide continuity of services and overcome problems of rigid systems, fragmented services, poor use of resources and problems of inaccessibility. The six activities that form the core of US case management are:

1. identification and outreach;
2. assessment;
3. service planning;
4. linkage with needed services – including mental health treatment, crisis response services, health and dental care, and housing;
5. monitoring service delivery;
6. advocacy.

In addition, core components and specific interventions related to clinical case management are listed in Table 5.1.

Functions of case management in the US will be an increasingly prominent part of mental health care in the future as attempts are made to balance cost, access and effectiveness. Resources of patients, families, providers and society must be managed in order to carry out these complex goals. However, important questions remain, including what the tasks of case managers are, who should be doing case management (what personal qualities and training are needed), to whom the case manager is account-able, and how the work of case management should be organised (Sledge et al., 1995; Vallon et al., 1997; Hall, 1998).

Nurses in the US have an opportunity to perform a variety of roles in case management. In particular, it allows nurses to assume direct care, super-visory and consulting roles while working with patients and families by:

- serving as their gatekeepers and facilitators in accessing the health care system;
- helping them make informed decisions about their health care needs:
- monitoring their health and human service plan of care;
- educating them to enhance their self-care ability.

In practical terms this means that the case manager has to have knowledge of social care systems and not just health ones, be able to access those systems on behalf of, and usually in the company of, the patient, have extensive personal contacts within different health and social care organisations and agencies, whilst at the same time using personal skills that enable them to establish both a trusting and an advisory relationship with the patient maintaining contact with them irrespective of the prob-lems that arise.

Consequently, the American Nurses' Association (1993) suggests that psychiatric and mental health nurses are highly qualified to function as both case managers and providers within managed care systems. They are positioned to have a maximum impact on the managed care of psychiatric clients because:

1. they are committed to improving access, quality and cost containment;
2. they understand prevention and wellness and know how to educate patients to improve health;
3. they know how to triage and assess the needs of patients;
4. they know how to accurately evaluate the necessity for in-patient admissions and continued hospital stays.

Thus there is great opportunity for nurses to expand their roles and develop new career directions by functioning as case managers who can address the physical and psychiatric needs of patients. This can include people with chronic mental illness as well as general psychiatric patients in

Table 5.2   Qualifications and functions of the psychiatric nurse case manager (US)

Desired skills/qualifications	Functions
Certification in Case Management	Needs assessment
Baccalaureate/Graduate/Postgraduate Education	Diagnosis
Physical and psychosocial assessment skills	Patient advocate
Empathy and enthusiasm	Family collaboration
Excellent communication skills	Liaison between physician, patient and reimburser
Negotiation skills	Access community resources
Consultation skills	Treatment planning
Critical thinking skills	Crisis intervention
Knowledge of evidence-based treatments	Health promotion
Creativity and flexibility	Relapse prevention
Attention to detail	Implementation of treatment plan
Computer literacy	Documentation
Data management	Monitoring of care
	Outcome measurement

Source: B. Greco and N. Worley (2001) 'Community psychiatric nursing care', in G. Stuart and M. Laraia (eds), *Principles and Practice of Psychiatric Nursing*. St Louis, MO: Mosby pp. 728–43.

out-patient settings (Rhode, 1997; Young et al., 1998). The desired skills and functions for the psychiatric nurse case manager in the US are listed in Table 5.2.

Assertive community treatment (ACT) was developed in Wisconsin in the early 1970s as a programme originally called Training in Community Living (TCL). It was created as a way of organising out-patient mental health services for patients who were leaving large State mental hospitals and were at risk for rehospitalisation. The original TCL model has been replicated in thousands of communities under names such as Continuous Treatment Teams (CTTs), Programmes for Assertive Community Treatment (PACT) and Intensive Case Management (ICM). This model programme provides a full range of medical, psychosocial and rehabilitative services. The essential elements of assertive community treatment are listed in Table 5.3.

ACT uses an interdisciplinary team-orientated approach that typically includes up to 10 staff members (nurses, psychiatrists, social workers, activity therapists) who meet regularly to plan individualised care for a shared caseload of patients who receive care for as long as they receive treatment. More than 75% of staff time is spent in the field providing direct treatment and rehabilitation. In a US survey of assertive outreach programmes, it was found that 88% had a psychiatric nurse as an integral

Table 5.3   Essential elements of assertive community treatment (ACT)

Organisation and delivery of services

1. Core services team
    (a) Fixed point of responsibility
    (b) Primary provider of services
    (c) Continuity of care and caregivers across time and functional areas
    (d) Low client-to-staff ratios

2. Assertive outreach and *in vivo* treatment
3. Individualised treatment
4. Ongoing treatment and support

Treatments and services provided

1. Direct assistance with systems management
    (a) Medications
    (b) 24-hour crisis availability
    (c) Brief hospitalisation
    (d) Long-term one-to-one clinical relationship

2. Facilitation of an optimally supportive environment
    (a) Assistance with meeting basic needs
    (b) Assistance with a supportive social environment
    (c) Assistance with a supportive family environment (psychoeducation)

3. Direct assistance with instrumental functioning (work, social relations, activities of daily living)
    (a) *In vivo* skills teaching
    (b) *In vivo* support
    (c) Environmental modification

Desired patient outcomes

1. Reduced symptomatology and relapse
2. Increased community tenure
3. Enhanced satisfaction with life
4. Less subjective distress
5. Improved instrumental functioning
    (a) Employment
    (b) Social relations
    (c) Activities of daily living

Adapted from M.A. Test (1992) 'Training in community living', in R.P. Lieberman (ed.), *Handbook of Psychiatric Rehabilitation*. New York: Macmillan.

member of the treatment team (Deci et al., 1995). ACT teams function as continuous care teams who work with patients with serious mental illness and their families over time to improve their quality of life. In effect, these programmes function as a community-based 'hospital without walls', providing a high-intensity programme of clinical support and treatment.

The role of the nurse in ACT differs from that of a general mental health case manager in that they are directly responsible for the provision of a therapy or forms of therapy. In addition to undertaking the social development and liaison work described earlier they are the primary therapist within the care package and, instead of referring clinical problems or responses to treatment on to other specialists, actually do this work themselves. This will also extend to giving medication. Herein lies the main difference between the two main types of case management: that which sees the case manager as essentially a broker (social model), and that which sees the case manager as a therapist (clinical model). The first of these is derived from the original social role, the second resulting from the general increase of nurses and health care workers within case management. The assertive component may apply to either because it simply denotes the intensity with which the contact between patient and case manager is exerted. The case manager will undertake to maintain contact with the patient no matter how resistive they are to such an approach, will keep working at a problem no matter how difficult it is and continue to support the patient irrespective of the opposition they may generate. The whole purpose of this approach is to firstly maintain contact to ensure that the patient is safe and secondly to uphold the integrity of the care programme. Both of these serve to tell the patient that they are important, have value as an individual and that the case manager is there for them no matter what happens. Keeping a patient out of hospital is the aim of such an approach, but only by giving that patient quality of life and dignity within the community. Numerous controlled clinical trials of ACT have been conducted with a wide range of people with severe mental illness, including patients with schizophrenia, war veterans, dually diagnosed patients and homeless people (Burns and Santos, 1995). These studies report that patients spent less time in hospitals and more in independent community housing. Their symptoms were reduced, their treatment compliance was increased and ACT costs were usually lower (Dixon et al., 1997; Mueser et al., 1998; Lehman et al., 1999). Furthermore, the Programme of Assertive Community Treatment (PACT) is recognised by the National Alliance of the Mentally Ill (NAMI) as the most effective service delivery model for community treatment of severe mental illness. As such, NAMI has launched a national grassroots effort called PACT Across America to educate people about PACT and to offer training, monitoring, certification and management services to those mental health agencies wishing to implement the PACT model.

The results of numerous studies have thus led researchers to believe that, for most patients with schizophrenia, case management is a necessary component of care (Lehman, 1998). The most frequently studied forms of case management, assertive community treatment and intensive case management have been associated with decreased psychiatric hospitalisation and housing instability, as well as moderate improvement in symptomatology and quality of life for persons with schizophrenia (Mueser et al., 1998). Furthermore, in a meta-analysis of the effectiveness of case management in the US over 20 years it was found that clinical case management and assertive community treatment were associated with reduced family burden, increased family satisfaction and decreased cost of care. In addition, both were equally effective in reducing symptoms, increasing clients' contacts with services, reducing drop-out rates, improving social functioning and increasing clients' satisfaction (Ziguras and Stuart, 2000).

Concerns in the US

Nonetheless, many believe that attention to how ACT has been disseminated and replicated in the US, and systematic studies of its adaptation within existing systems of care, are not adequate and more work needs to be done in this area. Furthermore, a concern of programme planners is that features of the ACT model may be either unnecessary or overly expensive ways of achieving adequate client outcomes. It has been noted that faithful adherence to these and other programme goals is not always easy in traditional systems. The specialised nature of ACT programmes makes them particularly susceptible to misunderstanding by administrators and clinicians trained in traditional treatment models and to policies that impede effective implementation. Even when administrators and clinicians are well-trained and eager to follow guidelines, problems with financing and organisational structures designed for traditional office-based treatment can lead them to deviate from ACT principles, possibly limiting its effectiveness (Clark, 1997). Thus, although well accepted in the US, clinical and service-based questions about case management programmes continue to raise debate in the field.

Case management in the United Kingdom

The US system of case management was piloted in the UK in the early 1990s but there have been the usual problems associated with transferring a care system or approach from one health care culture to another. These centre on the fact that care systems are usually organised differently and people have separate outcome expectations. In the UK the seriously mentally ill are a small group of individuals, defined by their regular use of care services and their consistent inability to cope, over time, with genuine independent living. So, too, case management services can be organised in several ways, but the usual configuration in the UK is for separate case management facilities to be added to existing, traditional community mental health teams, either as a discrete team in its own right or as additional team members. Ideally, health and social services should jointly fund them, although this has been slow to develop and currently most UK case management comes under the auspices of health care, though with health care reforms this is changing.

Clients are referred for case management for different reasons but usually because they are resistive to the approaches of traditionally organised community mental health nurses (CPNs), suspicious of what they see as punitive care from State-controlled mental health services (Ward et al., 2000), deemed to be at risk of falling through the net of existing service provision, or are in need of complex care for diverse long-term mental health problems (Renshaw, 1988). A case manager who may adopt various methods of meeting client needs handles recommended caseloads of up to 15 clients. Two reviews undertaken by one of the authors (Armstrong and Ward, 1966; Ward et al., 1999) show that very often UK case managers tend to adopt an approach to care dictated by their previous professional occupation. As over 90% of managers are from a mental health nursing background, their work tends to be primary contact and therapeutic in nature (clinical model), but others, such as those with a social work background, are more likely to use a brokerage approach (social model). However, research has also shown that many UK case managers use a combination of both models, adopting the practical work described above in the 'nursing role within case management' section as well as the treatment and therapy activities described in the 'assertive community treatment' (ACT) section.

Services provided by case managers in the UK are difficult to define because they are very much dependent upon the needs of the client. However, a broad spectrum of possibilities exist, including therapeutic befriending, support with activities of daily living, personal and social skills development, housing, State benefits, financial support, and recreational and social care. Within the UK system there is a recognition that clients admitted onto a case manager's caseload will remain there for a considerable period of time, if not indefinitely (Ward et al., 1999). The purpose of case management is to support individuals within the community, to enable them to attain the highest quality of life and to give them the support necessary to remain independent of in-patient mental health services. Although this could be said to be the intended outcome of all community mental health programmes, it should be remembered that clients receiving case management support will usually be those most damaged by their illness, generally requiring high levels of assertive contact with their case manager, possibly several times a day in some cases. They are also those most at risk of suicide, usually unemployable, and often without personal family networks to watch out for them. For many, case management is their only hope of sustaining any form of independent living.

Perhaps the greatest success of case management within the UK is that it has become a recognised part of the psychiatric vocabulary with practitioners perceiving it as something that actually meets patient needs, and researchers and senior members of the professions formulating viable research agendas to understand how it functions best.

One significant piece of work is that of the large project funded by the Kings Fund, the Sainsbury Centre for Mental Health and the Department of Health 'Working for London' (Kings Fund, 1999); this was primarily a combination of case management and ACT, which brought together distinct groups of workers, from health, social care, voluntary agencies and in one case probation services, into four separate projects. Using assertive outreach and replicating development work undertaken in the US, its purpose was to establish the effectiveness of multi-agency case management for the seriously mentally ill, with particular importance placed upon the support of those from ethnic minority groups. This sophisticated project was well funded, its participants properly prepared, and most importantly heavily involved users or ex-users of services. Although still not complete, it has already shown that case management cannot simply be added on to existing services. Rather it requires considerable planning, multi-agency collaboration and a discrete budget to give it a chance of success.

Finally, the UK system does have some strengths over its US counterparts which should, in theory, give case management an advantage. Services are largely in the public domain and therefore not dependent upon economic interests or insurance companies. Coordination and continuity of care through the Care Programme Approach (CPA) (Department of Health, 1990) and Supervised Discharge (Department of Health, 1996), particularly for the seriously mentally ill, is well organised. Additionally, comprehensive sectorisation of care, where the same team is responsible for both an individual's in-patient and community care, allows for a high degree of flexibility and response to changing client needs.

Concerns in the UK

Whilst accepting that research in this area is difficult to undertake and needs to be carried out over long periods of time, questions have been raised about whether clinicians are researching the right things in their attempts to establish the efficacy of case management. For example, Tyrer (2000) argues that much of the UK research into different forms of case management and specifically ACT has shown inconclusive results because investigators have been trying to identify which organisational method is best. Citing the work of Thornicroft et al. (1998), Wykes et al. (1998) and Burns et al. (2000), he concludes that research needs to concentrate on establishing the impact of evidence-based interventions used within client contacts, not the number of contacts themselves. Indeed the much-quoted UK700 Group (1999) itself established a rigorous project to explore the difference between standard and intensive case management without even considering what the two groups of case managers were actually doing with their clients.

Furthermore, doubts in the UK exist about its overall efficacy (McGrew et al., 1995), the effects it has on case managers (Kirk et al., 1993), the preparation of those case managers (Andrews and Teesson, 1994) and the absence of clients' involvement in both care programmes and services generally (Armstrong and Ward, 1996). Ward et al. (1999) also showed that little research had been done to explore the work of the case manager and that many so-called 'case managers' within the system were really traditional CPNs who simply had role changes without the necessary specialist preparation or a reduction in their caseloads. Thus, in the UK, it appears that there is still no conclusive evidence to augment calls for greater use of case management as it is currently being implemented.

Challenges facing case management

There are some differences as well as remarkable similarities in the issues and challenges facing the implementation of case management in the US and the UK. One must be cautious in evaluating the case management outcome research between the US and the UK because there are many differences in the systems of care. An overarching difference between the US and UK context is that of services versus programmes. Much of US research derives from self-contained, targeted programmes for specific patient groups with clinical and budgetary independence. UK research operates largely within the tax-funded monopoly National Health Service, though there are some exceptions to this. Furthermore, there is much wider acceptance of consumers, survivors of services or ex-users, being employed within the US system as case managers in their own right (Dixon et al., 1997). This is certainly not the case in the UK where ex-users of services are both less inclined to be involved in supporting State care services, and services themselves are reluctant to involve ex-users in any real way as part of the therapeutic process. In fact, as Burns and Priebe (1999) point out, there is excessive preoccupation with risk in UK mental health care and this extends itself to any genuine involvement of its patients or ex-patients.

Not every mental health care professional is convinced of the necessity to switch total care contact to community settings. Nor are they convinced that different therapeutic processes have to be introduced for different sub-groups of clients. Moreover, high proportions of staff are not adequately versed or familiar with intensive therapy techniques but provide standardised support within blanket services. Given these realities, there exists a philosophical resistance to the introduction of yet more complex and seemingly elitist care models.

So, too, a major challenge exists in the need to conduct research, which informs both case management models and the therapeutic processes used within these models. Evaluation studies are needed in which many outcome measures are employed that are culturally sensitive and locally relevant. The social consequences of community-based care, such as violence, disruptive behaviour and stigma, should increasingly be measured when mental health services are compared. Another major research agenda for case management is the need to disaggregate and evaluate individual components of complex interventions. One can therefore anticipate a new generation of research into case management that uses it as a vehicle to ask questions that are more precise and more difficult to answer, but that are likely to have more far-reaching importance for community mental health initiatives.

Tyrer (2000) acknowledges that there are cultural differences between countries that will interfere with the way services are designed, set up and managed. And Burns and colleagues (2000) have shown that studies in the UK have increasingly failed to replicate the significant advantages of case management over standard community care achieved in the early American (Stein and Test, 1980) and Australian (Hoult and Reynolds, 1983) work. But, Tyrer also states that, to establish clear evidence to support the investment in case management, researchers have to make every effort to investigate services that are configured in the same way as the successful ones in North America.

To further disseminate the benefits of case management programmes, distinct client groups need to be identified, funds need to be made available to support these services, providers need to be trained, supervised and supported as case managers, and planners must be given the evidence to support the use of case management. However, one crucial element of case management remains unaddressed: that of the role of nursing within whatever model is adopted. Case managers undertake essentially practical work. Much that is described within this chapter forms nothing more than the basis of that work with individual patient needs determining what should take place, when and by whom. It is a complicated and tiring role because the contact between patient and case manager is so intense. Yet despite this, very few studies have actually considered the day-to-day work of case managers and even fewer have explored their work within the clinical model as both providers of social support and therapist. This situation is further compounded because politicians and those who fund mental health services are unaware of the complexities of the challenges faced by case managers. Despite this it appears that both the UK and US governments are committed to case management, and with so much attention being paid to community care for the mentally ill, it is likely that the potential for a more robust approach to their care will continue to evolve over time. Hopefully this will include a better understanding of the training and support needed for case managers.

References

American Nurses' Association (ANA) (1991) *Nursing's Agenda for Health Care Reform.* Kansas City, MO: American Nurses' Association.

American Nurses' Association (ANA) (1993) *Position Statement on Psychiatric Mental Health Nursing and Managed Care.* Kansas City, MO: American Nurses' Association.

Andrews, G.A. and Teesson, M. (1994) 'Smart versus dumb treatment: services for mental disorders', *Current Opinion in Psychiatry*, 7: 181–7.

Armstrong, C. and Ward, M.F. (1996) *An Audit of the Training, Skills and Caseloads of Community Mental Health Support Workers Involved in Case Management.* Interim report No. 12. Oxford: National Institute for Nursing.

Atkinson, M. (1996) 'Psychiatric clinical nurse specialists as intensive case managers for the seriously mentally ill', *Seminars for Nurse Managers*, 4: 130–6.

Bachrach, L. (1981) 'Continuity of care for chronic mental patients: a conceptual analysis', *American Journal of Psychiatry*, 138: 1449–56.

Bergen, A. (1994) 'Case management in the community: identifying a role for nursing', *Journal of Clinical Nursing*, 3: 251–7.

Burns, T. and Priebe, S. (1999) 'Mental health care failure in England: editorial', *British Journal of Psychiatry*, 174: 191–2.

Burns, B. and Santos, A. (1995) 'Assertive community treatment: an update of randomized trials', *Psychiatric Services*, 46: 669–75.

Burns, T., Fiander, M., Kent, A., Obioha, C., Ukoumunne, B. S., Fahy, T. and RajKumar, K. (2000) 'Effects of case-load size on the process of care of patients with severe psychotic illness', *British Journal of Psychiatry*, 177: 427–33.

Burns, T., Fioritti, A., Hollaway, F., Malm, U. and Rossler, W. (2001) 'Case management and assertive community treatment in Europe', *Psychiatric Services*, 52: 631–6.

Case Management Society of America (1995) *Standards of Practice from Case Management*. Little Rock, AR: Case Management Society of America.

Chase, P., Gage, J., Stanley, K. and Bonadonna, R. (2000) 'The psychiatric consultation/liaison nurse role in case management', *Nursing Case Management*, 3: 73–7.

Clark, R. (1997) 'Financing assertive community treatment', *Administration and Policy in Mental Health*, 25: 209–20.

Deci, P.A., Santos, A.B., Hiott, D.W., Schoenwald, S. and Dias, J.K. (1995) 'Dissemination of assertive community treatment programs', *Psychiatric Services*, 46 (7): 676–82.

Department of Health (1990) *The Care Programme Approach for People with a Mental Illness Referred to the Specialist Psychiatric Services*. Joint Health/Social Services circular HC9023/LASS9011. London: The Stationery Office.

Department of Health (1996) *Guidance on Supervised Discharge after Care under Supervision and Related Provisions Supplement to the Code of Practice Published August 1993 Pursuant to Section 118 of the Mental Health Act 1983*. London: The Stationery Office.

Dixon, L., Hackman, A. and Lehman, A. (1997) 'Consumers as staff in assertive community treatment programs', *Administration and Policy in Mental Health*, 25: 199–208.

Doyle, A. (2001) 'Developing a successful nurse case management program', *Issues in Interdisciplinary Care*, 3: 115–19.

Firn, S. (1997) 'Developing nursing skills in an intensive case management service', *Journal of Psychiatric and Mental Health Nursing*, 4: 59–61.

Glettler, E. and Leen, M. (1996) 'The advanced practice nurse as case manager', *Journal of Case Management*, 5: 121–6.

Hall, J. (1998) 'State of the art case management', *Occupational Medicine*, 13: 705–10.

Hoult, J. and Reynolds, I. (1983) *Psychiatric Hospital versus Community Treatment: A Controlled Study*. Canberra: Department of Health.

Kings Fund (1999) *Working for London: A Joint Funded Project to Establish the Effectiveness of Multi-agency Case Management in London*. London: Kings Fund.

Kirk, S.A., Koeske, G.F. and Keoske, R.D. (1993) 'Changes in health and job attitudes of case managers providing intensive services', *Hospital and Community Psychiatry*, 44: 168–73.

Leff, J. and Trieman, N. (2000) 'Long-stay patients discharged from psychiatric hospitals', *British Journal of Psychiatry*, 176: 217–23.

Lehman, A. (1998) 'Translating research into practice: the schizophrenia Patient Outcomes Research Team (PORT) treatment recommendations', *Schizophrenia Bulletin*, 24: 1–12.

Lehman, A.F., Dixon, L., Hoch, J.S., Deforge, B., Kernan, E. and Frank, R. (1999) 'Cost-effectiveness of assertive community treatment for homeless persons with severe mental illness', *British Journal of Psychiatry*, 174: 346–52.

Marshall, M., Gray, A., Lockwood, A. and Green, R. (1997) 'Case management or severe mental disorders', in C.E. de Jesus Adams and P. Mari-J White (eds), *Schizophrenia Module of the Cochrane Database of Systematic Reviews*, Issue 2. Oxford: The Cochrane Collaboration.

McGrew, G.H., Bond, G.R., Dietzen, L., McKasson, M. and Miller, L.D. (1995) 'A multi-site study of client outcomes in assertive community treatment', *Psychiatric Services*, 46: 696–701.

Meuser, K., Bond, G., Drake, R. and Resnick, S. (1998) 'Models of community care for severe mental illness: a review of research on case management', *Schizophrenia Bulletin*, 24: 37–74.

Mullahy, C. (1998) *The Case Manager's Handbook*. Gaithersburg, MD: Aspen.

Nehls, N. (2001) 'What is a case manager? The perspective of persons with borderline personality disorder', *Journal of the American Psychiatric Nurses Association*, 7: 4–12.

Renshaw, J. (1988) 'Care in the community: individual care planning and case management', *British Journal of Social Work*, 10: 79–105.

Rhode, D. (1997) 'Evolution of community mental health case management: considerations for clinical practice', *Archives of Psychiatric Nursing*, 11: 332–7.

Rothman, I. (1992) *Guidelines for Case Management: Putting Research to Professional Use*. Itasca, IL: Peacock Publications.

Rubin, A. (1992) 'Is case management effective for people with severe mental illness? A research review', *Health and Social Work*, 17: 138–50.

Ryan, P., Ford, R. and Clifford, P. (1991) *Case Management and Community Care*. London: Research and Development in Psychiatry.

Sabin, J. (1998) 'Public-sector managed behavioral health care: I. Developing an effective case management program', *Psychiatric Services*, 49: 31–3.

Sledge, W., Astrachan, B. and Thompson, K. (1995) 'Case management in psychiatry: an analysis of tasks', *American Journal of Psychiatry*, 152: 1259–65.

Solomon, P. (1992) 'The efficacy of case management services for severely mentally disabled clients', *Community Mental Health Journal*, 28: 163–80.

Stein, L.I. and Test, M.A. (1980) 'Alternative to mental hospital treatment. 1. Conceptional model, treatment programme, and clinical evaluation', *Archives of General Psychiatry*, 37: 392–7.

Stein, L.I., Test, M.A. and Marx, A.J. (1975) 'Alternative to the hospital: a controlled study', *American Journal of Psychiatry*, 132: 517–22.

Thornicroft, G. (1991) 'The concept of case management services for mentally disabled clients', *Community Mental Health Journal*, 28: 163–80.

Thornicroft, G., Wykes, T. and Holloway, F. (1998) 'From efficacy to effectiveness in community mental health services. PRiSM Psychosis Study 10', *British Journal of Psychiatry*, 173: 423–7.

Tyrer, P. (2000) 'Are small case-loads beautiful in severe mental illness?', *British Journal of Psychiatry*, 177: 386–7.

UK700 Group (1999) 'Intensive versus standard case management for severe psychotic illness: a randomized trial', *Lancet*, 33: 2185–9.

Vallon, K., Foti, M.E.G., Langman-Dorwalt, N. and Gatti, E. (1997) 'Comprehensive case management in the private sector for patients with severe mental illness', *Psychiatric Services*, 48: 910–15.

Ward, M.F., Armstrong, C., Lelliott, P. and Davies, M. (1999) 'Training, skills and case-loads of community mental health support workers in case management: evaluation from the initial UK demonstration sites', *Journal of Psychiatric and Mental Health Nursing*, 6: 197–9.

Ward, M.F., Gournay, K. and Cutcliffe, J.R. (2000) *The Nursing, Midwifery and Health Visiting Contribution to the Continuing Care of People with Mental Health Problems: A Review and UKCC Action Plan*. London: United Kingdom Central Council for Nurses, Midwives and Health Visitors.

Wrinn, M. (1998) 'Case management faces opportunity and challenges', *Continuing Care*, 17: 16–21.

Wykes, T., Leese, M. and Taylor, R. (1998) 'Effects of community services on disability and symptoms. PRiSM Psychosis Study 4', *British Journal of Psychiatry*, 173: 385–90.

Young, A.S., Oscar Grusky, O., Sullivan, G., Webster, C.M. and Podus, D. (1998) 'The effects of provider characteristics on case management activities', *Administration and Policy in Mental Health*, 26: 21–8.

Ziguras, S. and Stuart, G. (2000) 'A meta-analysis of the effectiveness of mental health case management over 20 years', *Psychiatric Services*, 51: 1410–21.

SIX

Integrated care pathways: the 'acute' context

Julie Hall

Introduction

Demands to increase efficiency and effectiveness in the delivery of health care without compromising quality are commonplace. Following decades of mental health policy reform and directives to redress longstanding criticisms of institutional care, acute mental health services still face these same challenges. Professionals in this specialty are fully aware that in-patient psychiatric services have been at the centre of considerable debate: with perceived decline in therapeutic interventions, bed management problems, an absence of evidence-based practice and subsequent concerns over care experiences (Sainsbury Centre for Mental Health, 1998). Whilst sustained development has been illusive, acute in-patient services are now facing a time for social transformation fully supported by mental health policy (National Inpatient Task Group, 2002).

The modernisation agenda for acute in-patient mental health provision is described in the *Mental Health Policy Implementation Guide – Adult Acute Inpatient Care Provision* (NITG, 2002). Significantly this is the first United Kingdom mental health policy dedicated to acute in-patient mental health care. The guide considers the integration of acute provision with other mental health care systems, remodelling services and specific measures to overcome past problems. Integral to the modernisation process, care pathway arrangements are seen as a formula for ensuring that care experiences are built around the needs of service users, their families and carers. It is suggested that arrangements are needed to ensure that a service user's journey across services is negotiated, managed and agreed. Additionally therapeutic and organisational arrangements need to be determined, planned and coordinated.

Concerns over poor system coordination and lack of collaborative working are some of the issues which have prompted the increased use of integrated care pathways by mental health NHS trusts in the UK. The integrated care pathways developed, piloted and implemented by many mental health NHS trusts have shared philosophies with those suggested in the *Mental Health Policy Implementation Guide*. However, in many cases the use of integrated care pathways has become much more sophisticated, following trends in general medicine originating from the US. Over the last five years, organisations have been successful in developing integrated care pathways which determine

> locally agreed, multi-professional practice based upon guidelines and evidence where available, for a specific patient/client group. It forms all or part of the clinical record, documents the care given and facilitates the evaluation of outcomes for continuous quality improvement. (Riley, 1998: 30)

It is the use of such a tool for driving forward modernisation in acute care which is the focus of this chapter.

What are integrated care pathways?

Integrated care pathways are multi-professional care plans that provide detailed guidance for each stage in the care of patients with specific conditions, over a given period of time (Riley, 1998; Ellis and Johnson, 1999) and are used for day-to-day monitoring and quality assurance. Consequently, care pathways document the multi-professional care (including investigations, interventions, activities, assessments, etc.) required to achieve agreed outcomes; they comprise the elements shown in Table 6.1. The use of integrated care pathways began in the United States as a central component of their managed care philosophy. They evolved as a tool for improving fiscal accountability; integrated care pathways are also known as critical care maps, care paths, anticipated recovery paths and critical pathways.

By way of contrast, the adoption of the care pathway model within the UK is to ensure that the latest research is incorporated into clinical practice. By detailing multi-professional interventions, based upon the latest evidence guidelines and evidence patients receive the most appropriate care, delivered by appropriate professionals (Johnson, 1994).

Of course, not all patients progress as planned. As integrated care pathways define expected interventions within the delivery of care, variance from the pathway is therefore monitored and the causes analysed (Kitchener and Wilson, 1995). In turn, this enables a review of care

Table 6.1 Elements of an integrated care pathway

- Developed by multi-professional teams
- Plan of anticipated clinical care
- Includes measurable outcomes
- Defines standards of care to promote consistency and equity
- Follows a timeline (days, hours, outcomes, stages)
- System of multi-professional documentation
- Forms all or part of the clinical record
- Designed to meet local needs and constraints
- Incorporates evidence-based guidelines
- Uses variance tracking for day-to-day monitoring and review of performance
- Crosses organisational and professional boundaries
- Is never finalised and is a continually evolving tool

outcomes to help identify alternative strategies to improving subsequent care. Thus, evaluative action leads to:

- continual re-monitoring of care provision;
- a focus upon quality improvement;
- changes in the pathway;
- problem solving;
- improved risk management;
- individualised care provision.

Arguably, arranging care using a predetermined philosophy may seem illusive, impractical or inappropriate to some professionals. However, in services sporadically characterised by depressing portrayals of fragmented care experiences (Mind, 2000) the alleged benefits of integrated care pathways warrant further consideration by all stakeholders, and especially those charged with modernising acute in-patient services. The key benefits of care pathways are clinical effectiveness, evidence-based practice, risk management, interprofessional working and appropriate bed management. Notably, these issues have significant relationships to the current 'acute concerns' associated with acute in-patient services (DoH, 1999a).

Professional benefits

Integrated care pathways are described as an exceptional tool for monitoring patient progress and provision of a written criterion of care (Mosher et al., 1992). Critics of traditional care plans view care pathways as a timely replacement for outdated systems of planning and delivering nursing care. In replacing traditional care plans, pathways are said to simplify documentation, reduce duplication and enable the development of a multi-professional patient record (Johnson, 1994). Mosher et al. (1992) found that nurses using pathways reduced time that they spent on documentation by as much as 80%, affording them more time to spend in direct interventions. This is a desirable improvement in any care context, and important to acute in-patient care where nurses are often perceived as too busy to spend time with patients, often citing paperwork as the underlying cause (Whittington and McLaughlin, 2000).

Developing pathways also provides opportunities for professionals to clarify roles, responsibilities, interventions and resource utilisation, improving communication and collaborative working (Mullins and Wilson, 1994). This activity is timely and relevant to nurses in acute in-patient settings where evidence of effective interventions is beginning to emerge (DoH, 1999a; Institute of Psychiatry, 2001). The process of pre-formulating care provides a framework to review the evidence which supports this specialism. Hence, this is an ideal opportunity for teams to consider the interface between their traditional caring role, biological interventions, psychosocial developments and the expressed needs of service users.

Additionally, care pathway development provides the framework to review existing practice and care outcomes (Jones and Mullikin, 1994; Johnson, 1996). Critical examination of current practice should exist as a fundamental element of health care delivery. Implementation of clinical guidelines and continuous appraisal of care outcomes is integral to a quality improvement approach to care. Recorded variances as part of the pathway process provide information facilitating clinical audit and allow care to be individualised. Where variances are used as part of the audit cycle, variations from standards can be minimised and improvements to care can be rapidly adopted into practice and evaluated (Kitchener et al., 1996).

An agreed pathway of care provides direction, consistency and certainty. Pre-formulation enables health care professionals to proceed through agreed interventions without having to wait for ward rounds and consultations (Rasmussen and Gengler, 1994), aiding decision-making, reducing delays and duplication. This was demonstrated by New (1995) who outlined benefits where patients (with a shared diagnosis) are admitted to numerous clinical areas under the care of several physicians, receiving treatment from many professionals within one hospital. In this case the implementation of a pathway encouraged a system of controlled multi-professional care delivery which facilitated communication, the use of shared clinical guidelines and continuous monitoring. These same benefits can be realised in mental health services which span large geographical locations and where professionals move through different parts of services. Pre-formulation helps secure the continuity of services delivered; although this consistency does raise critical questions about whether pathways stifle individuality and autonomy (Laxade and Hale, 1995; Wilson, 1995; Hotchkiss, 1997).

Debates of task orientation versus individualisation are well documented. Sceptics suggest that variances do not allow enough individualisation, whilst Walsh (1998) contests whether traditional care delivery ever became individualised. Indeed, this view is corroborated in a recent study of acute in-patient mental health care where traditional care planning systems are described as generally failing to involve service users in decision-making processes (Anthony and Crawford, 2000). Advocates of care pathways, Hotchkiss (1997) and Kwan-Gett et al. (1997) reiterate that they are guidelines to care delivery, not rigid protocols, and therefore individualism rests in the control of the professionals themselves. Agreeing with this, Hall's (2001) study of a mental health care pathway pilot found that professionals did not experience constraints to their professional judgement. Professionals felt fully able to exercise professional decision-making processes. It was believed that an individualised approach to care is a personal philosophy which was not compromised by the implementation of a care pathway (Hall, 2001). Pathways, therefore, are no substitute for professional judgement and each situation warrants assessment as suggested in a professional's duty of care.

Organisational benefits

Evaluative studies by Coffey et al. (1992), Petryshen and Petryshen (1992) and Johnson (1994) agree that increased efficiency resulting from the implementation of pathways can reduce the length of stay for some conditions and lead to organisational savings. However, in the case of a mental health care pathway, Groves (1990) and Jones (1996) acknowledge that length of stay cannot always be an adequate measure of quality. Evidently in-patient stays have been criticised as too short to stabilise enduring mental health problems. Or conversely, discharge is delayed due to poor integration with aftercare provision. Additionally, length of stay cannot be a significant measure of cost improvement if overburdened community resources fail to cope with existing demand and clinical deterioration. Whilst pathways may be a vehicle for improving bed management arrangements they should not compromise clinical decision-making in determining length of stay. Neither will they alone redress the problems associated with the zealous reduction in psychiatric beds over the last decade. Demand for acute psychiatric beds currently exceeds supply (DoH, 1998, 1999a, 2000). Despite reducing length of in-patient stay through the

1990s, wards frequently exceed 100% occupancy. Although acute services consume two-thirds of mental health expenditure, access to vacant beds and intensive care provision remain poor (Shepherd et al., 1997). Integrated care pathways will without doubt increase the scrutiny into how beds are used.

Research by Fulop et al. (1996) and Shepherd et al. (1997) suggests that one-third of in-patients on acute wards can be more appropriately placed and that many crisis admissions are avoidable. Alternatives to admission are often not available or considered; however, these certainly need to be considered as part of the journey through services. In response, care pathways can encompass gatekeeping arrangements and care programme approach principles to stimulate swift and appropriate access and efficient discharge planning. Bed management problems imply poor integration with other services and a lack of clarity in the purpose of acute in-patient care (DoH, 1999a). Whilst recent mental health policies have claimed a whole systems approach, the interfaces between different elements of services are often poorly coordinated (DoH, 1998, 1999a; NITG, 2002). Care pathway development offers the opportunity not only to consider the role, aim and philosophy of individual teams, but also how they contribute to the whole care experience. Pathways which span professional boundaries (Anders et al., 1997) can enable in-patient services to be less isolated and devalued.

Legally it is suggested that pathways have the potential to reduce liability and enhance legal advantages (Forkner, 1996). Systems which improve communication, relationships, standards of documentation and collaboration are a welcome tool in reducing litigation. Maclean (1993) and Weingarten (1993) verify that the use of clinical guidelines has been shown to improve clinical outcomes, reduce error and increase effective practice. The study of a myocardial infarction pathway illustrates that where an integrated care pathway is adopted, patients are more likely to achieve the standards of care described than they were prior to pathway implementation (Johnson, 1996). A comparative study by Roebuck (1998) substantiates this, identifying improvements in 35 out of 36 audit outcomes where the outcomes were facilitated through the pathway. In addition, it was reported that the clinical area had experienced a 90% reduction in complaints. Cumulatively, these are indications of significant legal benefits which also help organisational drives to improve performance indicators.

Improved efficiency without the loss of quality is at the centre of the care pathway concept. Arguably the cost-saving aspects of managed care are also highly valuable to mental health care organisations. From an economic perspective care pathways clearly define the resources required during a specified episode of care. The specific and multi-professional nature of pathway documentation can result in the reduction of the duplication of services, consultations, investigations and interventions (Coffey et al., 1992; Petryshen and Petryshen, 1992; Laxade and Hale, 1995; Kitchener et al., 1996). Wigfield and Boon (1996) described the following benefits for organisations: enhanced multi-professional cooperation and collaboration, the constant review of clinical practice, evaluation of effectiveness, improved patient information, easier induction of new staff, less duplication of documentation and the ability to give high-quality information about services. Many of these benefits have been replicated into mental health pathway implementation (Hall, 2001). As poor communication accounts for many complaints it is worth noting that so many authors suggest pathways positively influence communication and reduce the incidence of complaints (Forkner, 1996; Petryshen and Petryshen, 1992; Wilson, 1997). Communication is improved as professionals report that they know what is expected of them and each other. They have documentation that is shared and facilitated through the pathway. The route of care can be easily followed to see what has been achieved and what is yet to be implemented. A named professional manages the pathway and information is easily accessible. This replaces systems where clinical notes are kept separately and never interact.

Influence upon care experience

It is implied that pathways reduce the likelihood of patient complications, enabling the effective utilisation of resources and increase patient knowledge and satisfaction. Impact upon the incidence of complications and infections has been widely disputed (Kwan-Gett et al., 1997; Holtzman et al., 1998). The impact of mental health care pathways upon recovery or service user satisfaction is also difficult to quantify, however. A significant benefit identified by Kitchener et al. (1996) is the early identification through variance of patients who are not progressing as expected. Individualised approaches to management of the pathway allow for early intervention where care must be revised and alternative interventions offered. Beneficial to acute in-patient care, this indicates relapse, poor adherence to treatment and clinical deterioration. Where such issues are identified this readily indicates that risk management or specific clinical measures are required.

Pathways are available to service users as an educative tool to help reduce anxiety and promote involvement. Complex pathway documents can be translated to service user and carer formats as seen in Figure 6.1. Their use informs service users of anticipated care and can demystify treatment (Mullins and Wilson, 1994; Rasmussen and Gengler, 1994). It

This information aims to clarify what will happen now that you are in hospital.

Your care is explained as a pathway which flows from admission to discharge.

The Smith Ward pathway shows examples of the care that you can expect to experience during your stay. It is not always 'written in tablets of stone' – care delivery does depend upon your needs, response to treatment and discharge plan.

The team here wants you to ask questions, to participate in your care and let us know how we can help you reach your goals. We hope this information helps to start off this process.

On your day of admission

Today, you and your carers (where appropriate) will become familiar with the ward and facilities. The nurse arranging your admission will show you around, where you will sleep, etc. He or she will explain to you arrangements regarding visiting, meal times, telephones, postal services.... All of this information will be given to you in the ward information booklet which you can return to later.

During your admission you will be seen by a doctor and a nurse who will begin your assessment by evaluating your health. Together you will begin to work in developing your plan of care. You will be encouraged to participate in this process as much as possible. With your permission your family or other significant people can be involved.

During your admission the doctor will ask if you will consent to a brief medical examination. This will only be done with your consent and is a routine part of hospital admission to assess your physical well-being.

On the day of admission you will be allocated a Named Nurse – this is the person who will then be responsible for coordinating your care arrangements during your stay in hospital. This arrangement involves a partnership with you, your carers (where appropriate) and other members of the multi-professional team. If there is anyone you wish to know that you are in hospital or if there is anything urgent at home which needs attention you should let the nurse admitting you know.

After you have been seen by the doctor and nurse they will discuss with you your immediate care. Your further assessment, care and treatment can begin here; this will be explained, planned and negotiated to meet your individual needs. This pathway has some further information about what will happen during the rest of your stay. Please read on when you are ready. Ask your Named Nurse or any other team member when you need help or have any questions.

The next few days focus upon assessment and beginning your treatment.

You will continue to work with the team throughout your assessment. During this time you can expect to ...

Figure 6.1 Extract of an integrated care pathway document modified for service users and carers

is hoped that service users who receive more information are increasingly involved in their care. Opening the dialogue about anticipated care aims to be enabling, offering a format for a partnership, relationship building and communication. Remembering that pre-formulation should not compromise choice this is a juncture for working in partnership. Exercising roles, relationships and responsibilities is significant to recovery. This collaboration can aid the careful integration of evidence-based practice and individualised recovery. There are warnings that the pre-formulated ideology of pathways can detract from patient independence and responsibility (Jones, 1996). The fact that treatment options can be forwarded by the service providers without user involvement suggests that emphasis can be given to financial considerations rather than needs. That the UK NHS trusts generally have a monopoly for the provision of acute mental health services has long been an issue of debate. It would be an immense concern if care pathways are developed primarily with an organisational or fiscal agenda and do not help to increase levels of inclusion.

The discourse about social control in acute care and the nurse–patient relationships cannot be divorced from the care pathway debate. Debating interventions during pathway development in forums brings to light issues of containment and coercion. Service users in the care pathway development process raise awareness about impressions of enforced care and powerlessness. Ensuring that all stakeholders are represented in pathway development positively influences pathway content and care processes. Care characterised by respect, empathy, time, normalisation and skilled interventions are underpinning philosophies for development. This ideology ensures that care pathways do not impede individualised care or contribute to the social distance between nurses and service users. As pathways propose some degree of standardisation; service users can expect at least equitable treatment and rising minimum standards. Ensuring a minimum standard may indeed improve upon past experiences characterised by lack of contact and active intervention.

Several authors propose that an increase in multi-professional collaboration leads to an increase in patient satisfaction (Mosher et al., 1992; Petryshen and Petryshen, 1992; Tucci and Bartels, 1998). However, often studies do not adopt any formal methodology to measure correlation between pathway use and a subsequent increase in patient satisfaction. Many evaluative studies are retrospective in nature and therefore the administration of patient satisfaction surveys as a means of measuring improvement is impractical. A notable exception is Stead et al.'s (1995) study of a surgical pathway which showed a 12% increase in patient satisfaction over two clinical areas following implementation. Unfortunately the low response rate (33%) limits the impact of the study's findings. As yet there are no studies in the UK regarding the impact of mental health integrated care pathways upon service user satisfaction. However, service user involvement in pathway development is an appropriate vehicle to secure representation in service development. Bryant (1999) acknowledges

> The creation of integrated care pathways may only count in our tomorrows, I suggest, provided they have real and meaningful reason for being in existence. They are not just being organized for the ease of professional workloads, fulfilling some managerial ego

trip and for reducing costs, but they are designed to really support and care for the patients travelling along its route.

In summary the claimed benefits of care pathways are the following.

- Improved multi-professional communication and cooperation.
- Reduction in duplication of services.
- Reducing length of stay.
- Increased patient satisfaction and reduction in complaints.
- Reduction in errors and enhancement of legal advantages.
- Improvement in quality outcomes.
- Development of practice based upon research, guidelines and national standards.
- Improved staff morale and job satisfaction.
- Less time spent on documentation.
- Development of multi-professional documentation.
- Standardised care delivery through preferred specific goals, interventions, investigations and treatments.
- Early identification of variance: i.e., complications/relapse.
- Variance analysis as a means of risk assessment and continual quality improvement.

Limitations and difficulties

Roebuck's (1998) account of the development of pathways in oncology suggests that the main disadvantage of the pathway process is the time-consuming nature of development, and the commitment of resources required through the change process. This scenario is already familiar to those charged with facilitating change in health services. A great deal of leadership, commitment and drive is required to ensure that changes in practice are embraced into day-to-day reality. Implementing change in acute in-patient care has to contend with the context of the environment and its problems. The difficulties experienced in maintaining minimum staffing levels, with nurses working well in excess of their contracted hours, impacts upon commitment. The quality of work life for nurses in acute psychiatry is poor (DoH, 1999a; NITG, 2002) and change should not appear as a burden. It is probable that staffing problems, high levels of stress and low staff morale contribute to a climate which mitigates against improvements in services. Development processes must be flexible and creative in an environment where meaningful change is difficult to sustain.

It is acknowledged that pathways are significantly easier to develop in cases where there is less variance in the clinical course of the condition between patients (Kitchener et al., 1996). Jones (1996) discussed the unpredictable nature of serious mental illness and how mental health pathways are likely to be complex to develop and implement. Immediate difficulties in care pathway development are posed by an indeterminate timeline which offers structure to the content. Clinical manifestation of mental health problems are unique and difficult to generalise in terms of duration. Indeed, many individuals experience complications or develop outcomes which do not correspond with the pre-planned nature of pathways. These groups may therefore be disadvantaged as their care episode will not be researched, planned or evaluated with the same scrutiny as those subject to care pathways. The absence of mental health focus in the care pathway literature substantiates this outlook. Jones (1996) argues that individuals with severe mental illness often require sporadic and sometimes lengthy hospitalisation, in which the planning and implementation of managed care is 'futile and wasteful of resources'. However, it can be argued that in the current state of high demand and reduced resources, warrants even more the strive for efficiency and effectiveness during any hospitalisation (Petryshen and Petryshen, 1992). Integrated care pathways are a fundamental tool for developing such a response.

Adelman (1998) recognises that professionals are duplicating the time-consuming exercise of developing pathways and suggests that a clearing house for pathways would reduce reproduction in numerous health care settings. The need for local adaptation to core pathways is seen as a potential way forward to avoid expensive duplication. This is supported by Anders et al. (1997) who have developed a care pathway for the acute management of hospitalised patients with schizophrenia.

In the UK the National Electronic Library for Health offers a database of care pathways in use and under development. This enables organisations to share their work, reducing duplication of effort across different organisations. Additionally, this provides a framework for benchmarking across organisations to compare current practices.

It has been suggested that there is a fear among health care professionals that pathways too easily indicate deficiencies in care. Variance reporting identifies when interventions and outcomes have not been delivered or achieved. The concern is that this information may then be used as evidence of a breach of duty of care (Hotchkiss, 1997). However, Hotchkiss (1997) believes that this fear has not been a reality in the US where pathways have been in use for a considerable time. Tingle (1995) suggests that where health care professionals can demonstrate that they have thought proactively about care delivery and clinical protocols then they should not be penalised for this. Where organisations have been able to demonstrate this consideration and proactive stance this develops a legal advantage. Some parties debate that exposure to malpractice will increase, however, if practitioners do not deliver pre-planned interventions without substantial justification (Hirshfeld and Ile, 1990). In reality this barely differs from the current position in the UK in relation to clinical guidelines and protocols. Not surprisingly the legal aspects of integrated care pathways are widely and critically debated in the US; similar implications under British law are indicated (Garnick et al., 1991; Moniz, 1992).

The mental health modernisation agenda

Within the National Health Service – a service with ambitions (DoH, 1996) – and the new NHS – modern and dependable (DoH, 1998) – the government emphasised the importance of a high-quality integrated health service organised around the health needs of individual patients, spanning traditional professional boundaries, and determining how patients' needs might be met over a period of time. As the mental health modernisation agenda pursues collaborative interprofessional systems, many current directives, initiatives and innovations have significant relationships with integrated care pathways.

1. **Integrated working**. Care pathways adopt a strong integrative philosophy and deliberately use teamworking and shared belief systems from the outset. The aim is to ensure that care is a collaborative endeavour, as teamwork is a vital accompaniment of care delivery. Care pathway development requires in-depth discussion and negotiation in order to develop a shared understanding of a patient journey. The multi-professional record improves access to information and develops understanding of different roles and contributions. Developing and using the multi-professional integrated care pathway strengthens interdisciplinary accountability for patient outcomes. Improved communication between team members is a consequence of professionals working from an agreed plan. Describing a seamless pathway of care and articulating expected interventions brings increased pressure to ensure effective care delivery. These interventions and expectations are clearly expressed in care pathway documentation – see the extract in Figure 6.2.
2. **User and carer focus**. Service users are the only stakeholders who experience the whole system of care. Refocusing care to follow this journey, rather than how services are organised, reflects the interests of those receiving care. It is acknowledged that the views of professionals alone rarely reveal the limitations of services with the clarity and recognition offered by those who use services (Heyman, 1995). Gathering the range of views illustrates not only the existence of

problems, but illuminates the process of care to show how and why limitations arise. Evolving over years or decades, services have often had conflicting or vague aims and failed to represent the views of all stakeholders (Rossi and Wright, 1977; Berk and Rossi, 1999). Stakeholder groups prioritise efficiency, democracy, choice and respect differently and care pathway development places service users central to re-designing services. Using a pathway approach aims for service users and professionals working collaboratively together. Specifying interventions and processes ensures that all involved are aware of anticipated treatment, and the contributions they have to offer.

3. **Risk assessment and management**. Risk assessment strategies can be appropriately built into pathway content, although most significantly it is the reduction in variation in practice which contributes to significantly reducing variations in care delivery and clinical outcomes. Clarification of specific goals, interventions, investigations and treatments have been effective in reducing clinical-based errors and ineffective practice (Coffey et al., 1992; Mullins and Wilson, 1994). Risk management is credibly associated with variance analysis (Kitchener and Wilson, 1995). As care pathways specify outcomes, any failure can be clearly identified. Deviations from expected recovery identify clinical relapse and deterioration. This specific information is used to facilitate decision-making and shape individual interventions. In the longer term, systematically collecting variance data is credible and reliable for developing changes in practice which are clinically led (Kitchener and Wilson, 1995). This enables organisations to identify interventions which are ineffective, or have not been delivered and why. This information is analysed to consider how omissions and errors can be minimised.

4. **Evidence-based practice**. Care pathways incorporate clinical guidelines, standards and outcome measures. Defining the interventions incorporated into the pathway inevitably involves asking clinical questions, then searching for and appraising the evidence. Interventions can be compared with the research and opinions offered by respected experts. This process enables all stakeholders to critically review what is offered in the context of local services and agreements. Integration of professional expertise, scientific enquiry and service user perspectives form the basis of pathway content. The UK National Institute for Clinical Excellence protocols and treatment guidelines play an obvious role in the indication of cost-effective treatments and care processes. The care pathway development model is therefore used as a system for enabling change and ensuring that evidence-based practice reaches fruition. This will only be felt where the pathway is formulated by benchmarking best practice, incorporating

national and local standards and the application of research evidence. Ineffective and dangerous practice as a consequence can be eradicated.

5. **Managing service availability**. Considering anticipated elements of care for a particular journey through services inevitably begins by defining who will use services. Implicated are the core aims of the journey and the outcomes to be achieved. Answering these questions implicates the nature and volume of how mental health services are targeted and used. Care pathways serve as an ideal opportunity to focus upon 'gatekeeping' arrangements – defining how services are accessed and upon what criteria. Additionally, mapping care journeys incorporates a critique of care processes – identifying delays, duplications, hold-ups and deficiencies. Pre-defining care to an extent affords opportunities to ensure that by consensus view measures are taken to avoid delays and meet targets. Unnecessary are waits for consultants' ward rounds before treatment decisions or discharge arrangements are planned or implemented. Professionals and organisations can exercise their obligation to justify the use of resources and demonstrate improved quality of care. This ethos is in tune with the Mental Health National Service Framework for Mental Health (DoH, 1999b) aiming to ensure equity of access to services and implementation of standardised protocols for major diagnostic groups.

6. **Clinical governance**. Care pathways enable organisations to target effective interventions to effect the greatest clinical benefit. Clear care processes enable efficient checks to establish whether professionals are working towards quality standards. As care pathways identify clinical interventions, timescale and anticipated outcomes they offer a succinct framework to measure effectiveness. Data for audit are collected as an integral part of documenting care delivery. Analysis of variation from the pathway is used to refine practice, update the pathway and inform organisations about service needs. Regular review of pathway content and supporting evidence base informs training needs and ensures that high-quality patient care is maintained. Organisations can collect data to establish whether outcomes are achieved over defined periods. This enables a journey of care to be measured in terms of length of stay and effect upon health outcomes. Not surprisingly, some stakeholders are suspicious of this viewpoint and perceive that their position and autonomy are threatened. However, as the structures and strategies to increase corporate responsibility rapidly grow, care pathways are a likely vehicle for refining clinical governance mechanisms.

7. **Organisational strategy and corporate philosophy**. Care pathways embody organisational strategy and translate corporate philosophies

into practice. A pathway which accurately reflects the activities of the multi-professional team incorporating clinical guidelines and research-based information is locally based reflecting the approach of the organisation (Kitchener et al., 1996). Defining local practice offers an ethos for change and development which can be owned by those receiving and delivering care. Securing professional practice and enhancing patient care is often the focus of nursing strategy, and care pathway implementation enables change which is context specific and has regard for the characteristics of the organisation. Studies of pathway implementation often indicate improved levels of professional satisfaction (DeLuc, 2000; Hall, 2001). This is fruitful for organisations which need to adopt an ethos of organisational learning. The opportunity to tailor the pathway to local resources and expertise affords flexibility and use of an audit tool to test outcomes and plan services. Using care pathways ensures that all service users accessing a specific service can expect to receive the same quality of care and fair access to appropriate professionals and services.

8. **Information for health**. The National Health Service Executive (NHSE) (1998) have described their momentous programme for embracing advances in information technology to benefit patient care. The programme acknowledges the importance of patient-centred seamless care systems supported by information technology. The underpinning philosophy is to share information and improve access to information for all stakeholders. Care pathways are embraced into the programme in collaboration with electronic health and patient records, seamless services and systems which cross organisational boundaries and the primary–secondary care interface. Pathways are viewed as integral components to clinical governance, audit and evidence-based practice. The UK National Electronic Library for Health care pathway database suggests that there have been few examples of electronic integrated care pathways in practice to date. However, software companies in the UK are following their US counterparts and developing electronic integrated care pathway systems espousing their impact upon quality improvement and cost-effectiveness.

Acknowledging the mental health modernisation agenda indicates the relationships between care pathways and specific policy perspectives. However, there are few approaches to organisational development or managing care which are able to embrace the plethora of current directives. Carefully entwined and influencing care pathway development are processes of accountability, advocacy, the politics of organisations and policy, and the quality of professionals involved.

Figure 6.2 Extract showing clear multi-professional expectations. Reproduced by the kind permission of Dr Karen Moody from the State Hospital, Carstairs, Scotland, UK

MEDICAL INTERVENTIONS – ADMISSION ICP		
Same day	*Date and sign*	*VARIANCE – Please tick box as appropriate, write reason for variance, action taken and final outcome*
1. Admission mental state examination completed	../../..	☐ LATE ☐ NOT DONE ☐ N/A
2. Ward copied with pre-admission report	../../..	☐ LATE ☐ NOT DONE ☐ N/A
3. Physical examination (including neurological examination and general medical history completed)	../../..	☐ LATE ☐ NOT DONE ☐ N/A
By Day 7		
4. Folstein MMSE completed	../../..	☐ LATE ☐ NOT DONE ☐ N/A
5. Admission bloods (LFTs, U&E, FBC + ESR, glucose, syphilis serology, TFT) taken	../../..	☐ LATE ☐ NOT DONE ☐ N/A
6. Preliminary assessment by allocated Consultant	../../..	☐ LATE ☐ NOT DONE ☐ N/A
At CTM		
7. Initial strategic review completed	../../..	☐ LATE ☐ NOT DONE ☐ N/A
8. CC scheduled for W8	../../..	☐ LATE ☐ NOT DONE ☐ N/A
By Day 14		
9. Previous psychiatric admission/prison files requested	../../..	☐ LATE ☐ NOT DONE ☐ N/A
10. Request medication history from pharmacy (if indicated)	../../..	☐ LATE ☐ NOT DONE ☐ N/A

Continued

| 11. Referred for neurology opinion (if indicated) | ../../.. | ☐ LATE
☐ NOT DONE
☐ N/A |

By Day 49

| 12. Admission history compiled and sent to ward | ../../.. | ☐ LATE
☐ NOT DONE
☐ N/A |

At CC

| 13. Patient referred to high dose antipsychotic patients to ECG clinic (if appropriate) | ../../.. | ☐ LATE
☐ NOT DONE
☐ N/A |

| 14. CC attended by Consultant | ../../.. | ☐ LATE
☐ NOT DONE
☐ N/A |

| 15. Carers attend to CC | ../../.. | ☐ LATE
☐ NOT DONE
☐ N/A |

After CC

| 16. Information about schizophrenia given to carer after CC | ../../.. | ☐ LATE
☐ NOT DONE
☐ N/A |

| 17. Diagnosis discussed with patient | ../../.. | ☐ LATE
☐ NOT DONE
☐ N/A |

NURSING INTERVENTIONS

Prior to admission	Date and sign	VARIANCE – Please tick box as appropriate, write reason for variance, action taken and final outcome
18. Pre-admission assessment completed	../../..	☐ NOT DONE ☐ N/A

On admission

| 19. Transfer docs available on admission | ../../.. | ☐ NOT DONE |

| 20. Notes available on admission | ../../.. | ☐ NOT DONE |

Same day

| 21. Pre-admission assessment report in MDT notes | ../../.. | ☐ LATE
☐ NOT DONE
☐ N/A |

Continued

22. Patient introduced to ward	../../..	☐ LATE ☐ NOT DONE
23. Patient assigned to keyworker	../../..	☐ LATE ☐ NOT DONE
24. Patient introduced to keyworker	../../..	☐ LATE ☐ NOT DONE
25. Admission profile completed	../../..	☐ LATE ☐ NOT DONE
26. At-risk register completed	../../..	☐ LATE ☐ NOT DONE
27. Care plan commenced	../../..	☐ LATE ☐ NOT DONE
28. NOK contacted successfully	../../..	☐ LATE ☐ NOT DONE
29. Patient with physical disability and minority groups referred to clinical nurse spec.	../../..	☐ LATE ☐ NOT DONE ☐ N/A
30. Risk assessment tool completed	../../..	☐ LATE ☐ NOT DONE

By Day 5

31. Information booklets i.e., patient info., hospital info., section info. and MWC info given to patient	../../..	☐ LATE ☐ NOT DONE

By Day 7

32. Assessment tools, identified and completed by keyworker	../../..	☐ LATE ☐ NOT DONE
33. NOK letter with clinical team, visiting info. and info about CC sent	../../..	☐ LATE ☐ NOT DONE

At CTM

34. Risk assessment discussed	../../..	☐ LATE ☐ NOT DONE

By Day 14

35. Referral to occupational therapy for assessment completed	../../..	☐ LATE ☐ NOT DONE

Continued

36. 11 point assessment ../../..	☐ LATE
completed	☐ NOT DONE

By Day 49

../../..

37. Substance use	☐ LATE
screening assessment	☐ NOT DONE
and initial summary	☐ N/A
report completed	

Mental health care pathways in the UK

Health care providers in the UK are showing increasing interest in the claimed benefits of care pathways. In 1998 the National Pathways Association in the UK had 452 recorded pathways under research, pilot, implementation or evaluation. Eighteen of these pathways had a mental health focus. The current status of care pathway development is indicated by the National Electronic Library for Health care pathway database. The database shows a significant growth in the use of pathways in all specialisms, with in excess of 25 mental health care organisations registering their integrated care pathway developments.

Reviewing the literature corroborates the slow but growing use of mental health care pathways in the UK (Jones, 1997, 1999). Care pathways have been used for a range of mental health-related diagnoses in the US. There are predominant accounts of the use of care pathways for patients with schizophrenia (Anders et al., 1997; Jones and Kamath, 1998). Published accounts of mental health pathway development in the UK have focused upon schizophrenia (Jones, 1999, 2000) and dementia (Hall, 2000, 2001). One multi-professional team described their perceptions of a dementia assessment care pathway pilot.

- Team members corroborated many benefits of pathways expressed in the literature; i.e., increased efficiency, role clarification, evidence-based practice, professionalism, improved teamworking, enhanced communication, easier access to information.
- The effectiveness of the pathway was viewed as dependent upon a number of variables – the team, the patient group and available resources. For example, when equipment or particular specialists were not available, care was no further enhanced. The pathway merely indicated the deficiency and during the period of the pilot the pathway did not effect any improvement when such problems occurred.
- Recording and examining variances had proved to be stressful and frustrating for individuals. Not accustomed to making known limitations

and deficiencies – this meant a cultural change which was uncomfortable to some team members.

- The team clearly described anxiety regarding the theoretical construction of the pathway, and how professional congruence and accountability can be accommodated. Should the pathway content follow an idealised process or one the team knew they could realistically implement? This posed the team some ethical, organisational and professional dilemmas.

- The team did not comprehend the pathway as unworkable or unsuitable for use in mental health. Individualised philosophies and professional autonomy prevailed where feasible (Hall, 2001).

Jones (2000) discussed implementation of a care pathway for in-patients with schizophrenia. His study followed an action research methodology and clearly documented the complexities of implementing care pathways in mental health settings. Much of Jones's (2000) account discussed the change process experienced during implementation and the subsequent difficulties which arose. Notably the difficulties experienced reflect the circumstances which have frustrated rational change in acute in-patient care. The ward used to implement the pathway exceeded 100% occupancy, had a high proportion of patients experiencing severe mental illness and had a significant staff turnover. Collecting the data over the period of a year spanning pathway development and implementation the findings are striking. Amongst the findings Jones (2000) described difficulty engaging and sustaining professionals' commitment to the use of the pathway. The pathway was felt to be too simple to reflect the care process involved and commitment to use clinical guidelines was poor. Contextual issues of poor morale and staff turnover mitigated against a culture which could sustain the conditions required to embrace the pathway as a working norm. Jones (2000) goes on to further discuss the environment and culture required to sustain healthy development. What Jones's (2000) study clearly indicated are the barriers to using care pathways in mental health settings (Table 6.2). Conducted in an acute in-patient setting this offers clear guidance to those seeking to develop care pathways and other sustainable change.

Developing integrated care pathways

Over the last decade models for care pathway development have evolved, and a general pattern can be established. This general pattern is represented as a pathway development model in Figure 6.3. Contributing to this

Table 6.2 Barriers to implementation of integrated care pathways

- Difficulty in representing complex, flexible and fluctuating care processes in an integrated care pathway format
- Incompatibility with the unpredictable course of mental illness
- Legal implications of poor compliance with documentation standards
- Lack of evidence-based guidelines
- Fear and reluctance to change
- Low staff morale and high staff turnover
- Indifference towards clinical guidelines and evidence-based practice
- Bureaucratic inertia
- Insufficient leadership, commitment, creativity and time
- Perceived conflict with the principles of individualised care

model significantly are the works of Ignatavicius and Hausman (1995), Johnson (1997), Stephens (1997) and Campbell et al. (1998).

Care pathway development begins by selecting a case type or client group. This is often determined by patient population, or high-cost, high-volume, high-risk and complex case groups. There are also indications that pathways have been developed for certain patient groups because of a high level of interest among professionals, or alternatively by organisations when it is realised that there are considerable variations in practice which affect clinical outcomes. Additionally where organisations have reconfigured their boundaries the fundamental rethinking about the way services are delivered adds to the impetus driving care pathway development. Development involves collaboration and representatives of all stakeholder groups working together. The time span for the pathway should be agreed. This may involve bridging the primary and secondary care interface and certainly spanning organisational boundaries. The time span determines where the pathway begins and ends. This enables the care to be mapped in hours, days, weeks or in phases or stages of treatment/intervention.

The pathway development team review the aims and outcomes of the service. These can be identified in terms of patient and process outcomes. It is often at this point that fundamental rethinking about the way services are delivered begins. For instance, considering the history of services, contemporary patient needs, the felt experience, flow rate, inputs, outputs and volume. Assumptions from the past are challenged; leadership and support for change is critical. Multi-professional collaboration and communication begins to develop integrated thinking and an agreed understanding of service provision. All stakeholders are involved in process mapping, identifying major steps and activities through the time frame. Also contributing to this mapping are patient diaries, focus groups and review of medical

Figure 6.3   Pathway development model

Stage 1	*Select a case type or client group.* This involves data collection to determine patient population, high-cost, high-volume, high-risk and difficult-to-manage case groups. The case type or client group can be determined through diagnosis, procedure, patient need or stage/phase of treatment. Indications for use may also be a high level of interest among local staff, or where variations in practice occur and affect patient outcome.
Stage 2	*Establish, develop and educate the authoring team.* Determine staff interest and secure support from the clinical setting, multi-professional team and service user/carer representatives.
Stage 3	*Select the time frame and parameters.* This determines where the pathway begins and ends. The time frame enables the care to be mapped in hours, days or weeks, or in phases or stages of treatment/intervention.
Stage 4	*Determine the goals and outcomes of care.* The pathway team must determine the goals and outcomes of care within the chosen parameters. These can be identified in terms of patient and process outcomes.
Stage 5	*Process mapping.* All stakeholders mind-map the major steps and activities through the time frame. Review of medical records to establish practice patterns. Consider problems and issues at each step. Include approximate time periods and parallel processes. Establish loops, complexities, roles and relationships.
Stage 6	*Search for evidence-based interventions.* Review the literature, established guidelines and national recommendations which influence the expected integrated care pathway.
Stage 7	*Analysis.* Critically review the care process mapped and steps for appropriateness and timeliness – determine roles, duplications, delays and added value. Compare current practice with established clinical guidelines and benchmark across other organisations. Identify key areas for pathway/service development.
Stage 8	*Redesign.* Redesign the process around the experience of receiving care. Revise processes in terms of coordination, preplanning and removing steps with no added value. Incorporate evidence-based interventions, extend roles and match capacity to demand. Develop, consult and review a sustainable, feasible vision based upon best practice.
Stage 9	*Map the anticipated care and write the pathway.* Mould together the corporate care pathway template, variance analysis system and prevailing clinical documentation.
Stage 10	*Review, consult and revise.* Pathway development team, clinical staff and organisation approval.
Stage 11	*Develop implementation plan.* Dissemination/consultation, staff education, establish champions in the clinical areas, pilot (3 to 6 months), monitoring to assess the level of completion and variance analysis (after 30 cases).
Stage 12	*Review the pilot, revise and fully implement.* Monitor and evaluate usability, content and influence upon outcomes. Revise where necessary and fully implement.

Stage 13	*Quarterly variance analysis.* Present data to identified members of the multi-professional team and organisation. Consider in light of the analysis review of clinical activity and care processes. Develop action plans and the pathway to address adverse variances.
Stage 14	*Annual review.* Revise and upgrade pathway content according to emerging evidence, variance analysis and organisational developments.

Note: Considering the evolutionary nature of pathway development it is acknowledged that this model is not an entirely linear process.

records to establish practice patterns. The approximate time, problems, issues and parallel processes at each step are identified. The NHS Modernisation Agency (2002) describes parallel processes as non-direct interventions that contribute to the patient journey; i.e., referral processes. Loops, complexities, roles and relationships are acknowledged.

After the focus, time frame, outcomes and mapping have been completed, there is enough data to identify keywords and search for evidence-based interventions. A thorough and critical review of the literature is completed. Established guidelines, systematic reviews, meta-analyses and national recommendations which influence the expected integrated care pathway content are identified. The pathway development team then critically review the process map. Each step is critiqued for appropriateness and timeliness – determining roles, duplications, delays and added value. Interventions are compared with established clinical guidelines and benchmarked across other organisations. This enables the process map to be re-conceptualised, identifying key areas for development. The process is then redesigned around the experience of receiving care. Processes are revised in terms of coordination and preplanning, and steps with no added value are removed. Evidence-based interventions are incorporated, roles defined and capacity matched to demand. A sustainable, feasible vision of the pathway based upon best available evidence is developed and disseminated for consultation.

The redesigned care process is moulded with the corporate pathway template, variance analysis system and prevailing clinical documentation. Each integrated care pathway has its own implementation plan which considers dissemination/consultation, staff education, establishing champions in the clinical areas, pilot duration, monitoring and variance analysis. The pathway is piloted then reviewed in respect of usability, content and influence upon outcomes. The pathway is then revised and fully implemented. Quarterly variance analysis is performed with data presented to specified members of the multi-professional team and organisation. In light of the analysis, clinical activity and care processes are reviewed. Action plans and the care pathway are developed to address adverse variances. An annual review to revise and upgrade pathway content according to emerging evidence, variance analysis and organisational development is recommended. Considering the evolutionary nature of change it is acknowledged that the care pathway development model is not an entirely linear process.

Implementation and evaluation

Successful developments in health care are underpinned by high-quality education and consultation. Similarly, care pathway implementation requires collaboration characterised by high quality innovative support and leadership. Significant to success is the Care Pathway Facilitator who fulfils a project management role. Local implementation requires proactive champions at practice level to provide local support and monitoring. Details of these roles are often indicated on the lead page of integrated care pathway documentation – see Figure 6.4.

Clinicians provide the crucial care management role, implementing the pathway. This is a named individual responsible for coordinating the journey through the care pathway, facilitating the pathway continuum (controlling, coordinating, delegating and guiding care). This is suggested to enhance nurses' feelings of autonomy and professionalisation. Mosher et al. (1992), Johnson (1994), Roebuck (1998) and Zacharias et al. (1998) suggest that nurses implementing pathways can experience increased role satisfaction and a sense of empowerment.

Campbell et al. (1998: 135) describe that professionals

using care pathways should be encouraged to:

(1) Follow the integrated care pathway for every patient with the chosen condition.
(2) Complete integrated care pathway documentation, signing for key elements of care provided as they are carried out.
(3) Be free to deviate from the care specified in the integrated care pathway provided they justify the deviation and enter this in the variance sheet.
(4) Take appropriate action when the integrated care pathway identifies patients whose progress is less good than expected or faster than expected.
(5) Ensure that patients understand the care pathway as it relates to them, and allow them access to the integrated care pathway.
(6) Variance sheets should be inspected regularly to identify common reasons why the integrated care pathway was not followed. This should lead to discussion within the team and regular updating of the integrated care pathway when appropriate.

Figure 6.4　Integrated care pathway for acute adult admission & assessment

INTEGRATED CARE PATHWAY FOR ACUTE ADULT ADMISSION & ASSESSMENT	Lincolnshire Partnership NHS Trust

This Integrated Care Pathway is for individuals admitted to acute inpatient services. It is intended to guide admission and assessment ensuring that a service user's journey is negotiated, managed and agreed. As inpatient care is implicitly a request for urgent/intensive intervention there needs to be clarity regarding inputs and interventions required and how they will be delivered. Wherever possible interventions are based upon evidence and best practice. It is essential that the expectations of the individual service user are addressed as part of the overall care plan.

1. PERSONAL DETAILS

Name & Date of Birth: *(affix patient ID label)*	Ward: Unit/Location: Admission Date: Discharge Date:

Overall Objectives of this care pathway are to
- To initiate a therapeutic relationship and provide prompt expert assessment of individual needs
- Ensure effective care planning, co-ordinated care and risk management; user and carer involvement and communication
- Provide effective, evidence based interventions to help recovery
- Establish effective liaison and ensure that appropriate and necessary treatments and services are offered

Sources and evidence which inform the content of this pathway are;
DALE. M., DEMPSEY. K., ELLIS. J., O'HARE. J., STANBURY. C. & STODDART. Y. (2002). Getting Better Together – Reflections on the Mental Health Collaborative. Northern Centre for Mental Health; Durham
DEPARTMENT OF HEALTH. (2002). Mental Health Policy Implementation Guide – Adult Acute Inpatient Care Provision. Department of Health; London
STANDING NURSING & MIDWIFERY ADVISORY COMMITTEE. (1999). Mental Health Nursing – Addressing Acute Concerns. Department of Health; London

Instructions for use:

Before writing in this Integrated Care Pathway, please ensure you have signed the signature sheet (overleaf). When using this document please ensure that you date, time and sign against each activity when it has been completed. It is important to remember that the aim of the Integrated Care Pathway (ICP) is to ensure the most appropriate care is given at the correct time.

If an activity outlined in the ICP has not, for whatever reason, been completed then this must be shown as a variance. The variance record sheet should then be completed (page 29 & 30)

Continued

If further action needs to be taken, e.g. the intervention needs to be repeated, then use the blank spaces in the appropriate time frame of the ICP to record this. To view an example of a completed ICP please read the ICP file which is in your ward/area. These blank spaces can also be used to add interventions which are deemed appropriate for that person but are not already in the ICP. These additions should also be recorded as a variance.

It remains each professional's responsibility to ensure that practice is safe. This ICP is not a replacement for experienced clinical judgement and inter-disciplinary discussions. If you require further information please contact your Care Pathway Lead, Clinical Team Leader or Care Pathway Manager.

Variance analysis is critical to successful implementation. A variance is any digression from the planned pathway. Variances are recorded contemporaneously throughout the pathway either in a space alongside the interventions (see Figure 6.2) or in tables at the foot of each page; for example:

Variance tracking		
Data and time	**Variance: reason and action taken**	**Signature**

These may indicate positive factors – i.e., rapid clinical improvement and early discharge – or where interventions are not delivered or outcomes have not been achieved. The latter helps to indicate clinical deterioration. It has been found that recording and examining variances can be stressful and frustrating for individuals (Hall, 2001). Professionals are not accustomed to making known what they are unable to deliver or identifying the interventions that they cannot facilitate due to lack of time or skills. Professionals are uneasy with making known these factors, and organisations need to be supportive rather than critical towards this information. There are often training and resource implications associated with significant variance trends. Variance analysis makes known recruitment and retention difficulties and longstanding performance problems – these data can be organisationally enlightening although politically difficult. Variance data have an objectivity which are difficult to dispute and credibility for teams who wish to cite evidence in claims for increased resources.

Recording variances involves identifying what the variance is, the cause of the variance and any action plan needed to address the variance. The reasons why practice digresses from the integrated care pathway can be examined to identify variation in professional standards. This information is used for both day-to-day clinical management and continuous quality improvement. Over a period of time these data can be examined to establish trends, develop action plans and improve practice. For example, Hall (2000) found that group assessments by occupational therapists for those newly admitted for dementia assessment were often not completed and recorded as a variance. The variance in most cases was caused by high levels of confusion associated with a recent change in environment. A simple action plan was developed to ensure that this assessment was offered on an individual rather than group basis in the future. This enabled the occupational therapists to respond to the communication needs of the individual and complete the assessment without the added stress of a group-work situation. This is a simple but practical example of how variance analysis reports and effects upon outcomes are discussed by a multi-professional team. From this process an action plan is developed and practice reviewed.

Despite mainly favourable opinions of care pathways, many evaluative case-studies appear weak in research design and statistical rigour. Research into mental health care pathways in the UK in the future may be able to exploit links to the mental health minimum dataset and the Health of the Nation Outcomes Scales to aid evaluation. Whilst the literature does not invalidate the concept of care pathways, quantitative studies would be more widely accepted with the exposure of a control group which is absent from many studies. Evidence to date is largely anecdotal and does not enable conclusive evaluation of the effects of care pathways. There are no systematic reviews of the use of mental health care pathways. Many studies are deficient in statistical evaluation of cost reduction or effect upon length of stay. Those which demonstrate a more rigorous statistical design demonstrate only a small effect upon the use of resources and little effect upon clinical outcome (Kwan-Gett et al., 1997; DeLuc, 2000). There are few examples of trials without randomisation, single group pre-post, cohort, time-series or matched-case control studies. Many favourable reports rely upon narrative evidence, and an absence of rigorous analysis of data fails to substantiate anecdotal claims. Irrespectively, interest in care pathways remains high and gathers momentum, and therefore the potential benefits of implementation continue to warrant rigorous evaluation.

Integrated care pathways: nurses and practice development

Few would argue against the need for professional development and social transformation in acute mental health in-patient services. Characteristics of

Table 6.3   Factors which influence successful implementation

- Successful selling of the benefits to all stakeholders
- User involvement in pathway development
- Working practices amenable to shared systems of record keeping
- Clear information-sharing agreements across organisational boundaries
- Organisational and local commitment to integrated care pathways
- Availability of clinical guidelines and evidence
- Integration with electronic recording systems
- Involvement and ownership of staff on the ground
- Time, good working relationships and energy
- High levels of support during implementation (provided by the care pathway facilitator and local champions)
- Training in the use of documentation and new interventions

this situation can be seen as socially rooted, manifesting themselves in low morale and decline in therapeutic interactions (professionally known as acute concerns). These social issues are not unlike those which underpinned Lewin's (1946) early action research theories. Similar to action research, care pathway development requires a process of collaborative investigation, which develops knowledge to solve problems and bring about change (Hart and Bond, 1995). Care pathway development is situational and firmly rooted in human values and behaviours. The social nature of change required to respond to acute concerns is consistent with how care pathways are developed. It is known that economic strains, re-organisation and cost cutting have increased demands upon nurses (Hummelvoll and Severinsson, 2001). Resulting from drives for increased efficiency and lack of organisational support, burnout, professional inadequacy and exhaustion amongst nurses is high. Nurses in acute services require support to develop practice, and frameworks to support this have been lacking. Studies of acute in-patient care indicate that nurses do want to develop their practice (Bray, 1999; Hummelvoll and Severinsson, 2001). Perhaps illusive has been the focus, direction and structure to engage with the optimism and enthusiasm that are evident. There are a number of factors that influence the successful implementation of integrated care pathways (Table 6.3). Studying these factors will indicate levels of readiness in the particular clinical setting and where impetus will be needed for success.

Care pathways offer nurses in acute care the opportunity to increase their understanding of the nature of their situation and validate their practice. This approach is rooted in culture, group process, democracy and collaborative change (Adelman, 1993). Development can therefore be grounded in the context of acute mental health services. Process mapping identifies problems, innovations and solutions rooted in everyday practice. The underlying causes, assumptions and beliefs which influence current problems are revealed and analysed, and change often means challenging basic assumptions (Hendry, 1996). Care pathways, whilst having managerial-driven ethos, enable nurses to have a voice in changing acute mental health services through a more contextual approach. For the necessary changes to occur, organisations and professionals are required to reconstruct their reality and take responsibility for their role in the situation.

Summary

This chapter set out to consider the use of integrated care pathways to respond to 'acute concerns'. Examining the current acute context and mental health modernisation agenda indicates how closely care pathways are in tune with developments. Reviewing the literature indicates how a growing although largely anecdotal evidence base supports the use of integrated care pathways in mental health. The potential benefits and limitations of their use in the context of mental health care have been discussed. As an approach to developing change in acute in-patient service care pathways can integrate the dimensions of culture, challenge basic assumptions and potentially effect some acute concerns. More importantly they offer the opportunity to embrace acute care forums and truly map the care processes to enhance the felt experience of service users. This responds to the social nature of change that is needed in acute mental health services. For nurses this does not ignore morale or philosophy, but works to increase professionalisation and develop practice. With organisational support there is a significant likelihood of bringing together the agendas of practitioners, managers, service users and policy makers through change developed and owned in the clinical setting. The key advantage of integrated care pathways in this context is assisting the facilitation of change which has eluded many acute in-patient services for too long.

References

Adelman, C. (1993) 'Kurt Lewin and the origins of action research', *Educational Action Research*, 1 (1): 7–34.

Adelman, S.H. (1998) *A Proposed New Clearing House for Clinical Pathways* (http//www.hss.org/clinpath.html).

Anders, R.L., Tomai, J.S., Clute, R.M., and Olson, T. (1997) 'Development of a scientifically valid co-ordinated care path', *JONA*, 5 (27): 45–52.

Anthony, P. and Crawford, P. (2000) 'Service user involvement in care planning: the mental health nurses' perspective', *Journal of Psychiatric and Mental Health Nursing*, 7: 425–34.

Berk, R.A. and Rossi, P.H. (1999) *Thinking about Program Evaluation 2*. London: Sage.

Bray, J. (1999) 'An ethnographic study of psychiatric nursing', *Journal of Psychiatric and Mental Health Nursing*, 6: 297–305.

Bryant, L. (1999) *Paper Presented at the National Care Pathways Association Annual Conference 22nd July 1999*. York: National Care Pathways Association.

Campbell, H., Hotchkiss, R., Bradshaw, N. and Porteous, M. (1998) 'Integrated care pathways', *British Medical Journal*, 316: 113–37.

Coffey, R.J., Richards, J.S., Remmert, C.S., LeRoy, S.S., Schoville, R.R. and Baldwin, P.J. (1992) 'Introduction to critical paths', *Quality Management in Health Care*, 1 (1): 45–54.

DeLuc, K. (2000) 'Care pathways: an evaluation of their effectiveness', *Journal of Advanced Nursing*, 32 (2): 485–96.

Department of Health (1996) *The National Health Service – A Service with Ambitions*. London: The Stationery Office.

Department of Health (1998) *The New NHS – Modern and Dependable*. London: The Stationery Office.

Department of Health (1999a) *Mental Health Nursing: Addressing Acute Concerns*. London: The Stationery Office.

Department of Health (1999b) *The National Service Framework for Mental Health*. London: The Stationery Office.

Department of Health (2000) *The NHS Plan*. London: The Stationery Office.

Ellis, B.W. and Johnson, S. (1999) 'The care pathway – a tool to enhance clinical governance', *British Journal of Clinical Governance*, 4 (2): 61–71.

Forkner, D.J. (1996) 'Clinical pathways: benefits and liabilities', *Nursing Management*, 27: 35–8.

Fulop, N.J., Koffman, J., Carson, S., Robinson, A., Pashley, D. and Coleman, K. (1996) 'The use of acute psychiatric beds: a point prevalence survey on North and South Thames regions', *Journal of Public Health Medicine*, 18: 207–16.

Garnick, D.W., Hendricks, A.M. and Brennan, T.A. (1991) 'Can practice guidelines reduce the number and costs of malpractice claims?', *JAMA*, 266: 2856–9.

Groves, T. (1990) 'The future of community care', *British Medical Journal*, 300: 923–4.

Hall, J. (2000) 'Establishing an integrated care pathway within an organic inpatient assessment service', *CPD Bulletin Old Age Psychiatry*, 2 (1): 3–6.

Hall, J. (2001) 'A qualitative survey of staff responses to an integrated care pathway pilot study in a mental healthcare setting', *NT Research*, 6 (3): 696–705.

Hart, E. and Bond, M. (1995) *Action Research for Health and Social Care – A Guide to Practice*. Buckingham: Open University Press.

Hendry, C. (1996) 'Understanding and creating whole organizational change through learning theory', *Human Relations*, 49 (5): 621–41.

Heyman, B. (1995) *Researching User Perspectives on Community Healthcare*. London: Chapman & Hall.

Hirshfeld, E.B. and Ile, M.L. (1990) 'Practice parameters – the legal implications', *The Internist*, 31: 5.

Holtzman, J., Bjerke, T. and Kane, R. (1998) 'The effects of clinical pathway for renal transplant on patient outcomes and length of stay', *Medical Care*, 6: 826–34.

Hotchkiss, R. (1997) 'Integrated care pathways', *NT Research*, 2 (1): 30–7.

Hummelvoll, J.K. and Severinsson, E. (2001) 'Coping with everyday reality: mental health professionals' reflections on the care provided in an acute psychiatric ward', *Australian and New Zealand Journal of Mental Health Nursing*, 10: 156–66.

Ignatavicius, D. and Hausman, K. (1995) *Clinical Pathways for Collaborative Practice*. London: Saunders.

Institute of Psychiatry (2001). 'Inpatient care for mental health problems: a review of research and identification of researchable questions'. Unpublished, Health Services Research Department, Institute of Psychiatry, London.

Johnson, S. (1994) 'Patient focused care without the upheaval', *Nursing Standard*, 8: 20–3.

Johnson, S. (1996) 'Multi-professional pathways of care series – The National Pathway User Group', *Healthcare Risk Report*, 11–12 February.

Johnson, S. (1997) *Pathways of Care*. London: Blackwell Science.

Johnson, S. and Burall, K. (1996) 'Pathway to the heart', *Nursing Management*, 2 (4): 24–5.

Jones, A. (1996) 'Managed care: length of stay as a measure of quality', *Mental Health Nursing*, 16 (6): 12–13.

Jones, A. (1997) 'Managed care strategy for mental health services', *British Journal of Nursing*, 6 (10): 564–8.

Jones, A. (1999) 'Pathways of care in the inpatient treatment of schizophrenia: an experimental project', *Mental Health Care*, 2 (6): 194–7.

Jones, A. (2000) 'Implementation of hospital care pathways for patients with schizophrenia', *Journal of Nursing Management*, 8: 215–25.

Jones, A. and Kamath, P. (1998) 'Issues for the development of care pathways in mental health services', *Journal of Nursing Management*, 6 (2): 87–94.

Jones, R.A. and Mullikin, C.W. (1994) 'Collaborative care: pathways to quality outcomes', *Journal of Healthcare Quality*, 16 (4): 10–13.

Kitchener, D. and Wilson, J. (1995) 'Multi-professional pathways of care series – analysis of variance in patients', *Healthcare Risk Report*, 16–17 September.

Kitchener, D., Davidson, C. and Burnard, P. (1996) 'Integrated care pathways: effective tools for continuous evaluation of clinical practice', *Journal of Evaluation of Clinical Practice*, 2 (1): 65–9.

Kwan-Gett, T., Lozano, P., Mullin, K. and Marcuse, E.K. (1997) 'One year experience with an inpatient asthma clinical pathway', *Archives of Paediatric and Adolescence Medicine*, 151: 684–9.

Laxade, S. and Hale, C.A. (1995) 'Managed care 1: an opportunity for nursing', *British Journal of Nursing Management*, 4 (5): 290–5.

Lewin, G.W. (1946) 'Action research and minority problems', in G.W. Lewin (ed.), *Resolving Social Conflicts: Selected Papers on Group Dynamics*. New York: Harper & Row. pp. 201–20.

Maclean, D. (1993) *Clinical Guidelines: A Report to the Scottish Office*. London: HMSO.

Mind (2000) *Environmentally Friendly? Patients' Views of Conditions on Psychiatric Wards*. London: Mind.

Moniz, D.M. (1992) 'The legal danger of written protocols and standards of practice', *Nurse Practitioner*, 18: 9.

Mosher, C., Cronk, P., Kidd, A., McCormick, P., Stockton, S. and Sulla, C. (1992) 'Upgrading practice with critical pathways', *American Journal of Nursing*, 92 (1): 41–4.

Mullins, E. and Wilson, J. (1994) 'Medical care paths as part of an integrated organisational strategy', *Advisory*, 4–6 December.

National Inpatient Task Group (NITG) (2002) *Mental Health Policy Implementation Guide – Adult Acute Inpatient Care Provision*. London: Department of Health.

New, T. (1995) 'On the right path', *Health Service Journal*, 105, 5 October, p. 28.

NHSE (1998) *Information for Health*. Wetherby: Department of Health Publications.

NHS Modernisation Agency (2002) *Improvement Leaders' Guide to Process Mapping and Redesign*. London: The Stationery Office.

Petryshen, P.R. and Petryshen, P.M. (1992) 'The case management model: an innovative approach to the delivery of patient care', *Journal of Advanced Nursing*, 17: 1188–94.

Rasmussen, N. and Gengler, T. (1994) 'Clinical pathways the route to better communication', *Nursing*, 24 (2): 47–9.

Riley, K. (1998) 'Paving the way', *Health Service Journal*, 108: 30–1.

Roebuck, A. (1998) 'Critical pathways: an aid to practice', *Nursing Times*, 94 (26): 50–1.

Rossi, P.H. and Wright, S.R. (1977) 'Evaluation research – and assessment of theory, practice and politics', *Evaluation Quarterly*, 1 (1): 5–53.

Sainsbury Centre for Mental Health (SCMH) (1998) *Acute Problems: A Survey of the Quality of Care in Acute Psychiatric Wards.* London: Sainsbury Centre for Mental Health.

Shepherd, G., Beadsmore, A., Moore, C. and Muijen, M. (1997) 'Relationship between bed use, social deprivation and overall bed availability in adult psychiatric units and alternative residential options: a cross-sectional survey, one day census and staff interviews', *British Journal of Psychiatry*, 3 (14): 262–6.

Stead, L., Arthur, C., Cleary, A. and Wilson, J. (1995) 'Multi-professional pathways of care series – do multi-professional pathways affect patient satisfaction?', *Healthcare Risk Report*, 13–14 November.

Stephens, R. (1997) 'Setting up pathways in mental health', in J. Wilson (ed.), *Integrated Care Management – The Path to Success.* Oxford: Butterworth-Heinemann.

Tingle, J. (1995) 'Clinical protocols and the law', *Nursing Times*, 91 (29): 27–8.

Tucci, R.A. and Bartels, K.L. (1998) 'Ovarian cancer surgery: a clinical pathway', *Clinical Journal of Oncology Nursing*, 2 (2): 65–6.

Walsh, M. (1998) *Models and Critical Pathways in Clinical Nursing.* London: Baillière Tindall.

Weingarten, S. (1993) 'Reducing lengths of stay for patients hospitalised with chest pain using medical practice guidelines and opinion leaders', *American Journal of Cardiology*, 1: 15–27.

Whittington, D. and McLaughlin, C. (2000) 'Finding time for patients: an exploration of nurses' time allocation in an acute psychiatric setting', *Journal of Psychiatric and Mental Health Nursing*, 7 (3): 259–68.

Wigfield, A. and Boon, E. (1996) 'Critical care pathway development: the way forward', *British Journal of Nursing*, 5 (12): 732–5.

Wilson, J. (1995) 'Multi-professional pathways of care: a tool for minimising risk', *British Journal of Healthcare Management*, 1 (14): 720–2.

Wilson, J. (1997) 'Integrated care management', *Nursing Management*, 4 (7): 18–19.

Zacharias, S., Rodriguez-Garcia, A., Honz, N. and Hooper, C. (1998) 'Development of an alcohol withdrawal clinical pathway: an interdisciplinary process', *Journal of Nursing Care Quality*, 12 (3): 9–18.

SEVEN

Risk assessment and management in acute mental health care

David Duffy, Mike Doyle and Tony Ryan

Introduction

Types of risk

As an area of practice the management of risk in the mental health field has received considerable attention for a decade or so (see, for example, Monahan and Steadman, 1994; Alberg et al., 1996; Moore, 1996; Morgan, 1998; Prins, 1999; Ryan, 1999). The risk management literature is dominated by work on the risks of violence and homicide on the one hand and the management of self-harm and suicide on the other. While this chapter will address these areas it is also worth recognising that these are not the only risks people with mental health needs face and pose. Working with people in an in-patient setting may provide opportunities that relate to the management of other forms of risk and also support service users to develop the ways in which they and their informal carers can manage risk for themselves in the future.

We know that people with mental health needs are over-represented among those who find themselves homeless (Bines, 1994; Crisis, 1999; Housing Service Agency, 1999), imprisoned (Singleton et al., 1998) and unemployed (Labour Force Survey, 1997/8). While housing and employment issues, for example, might not be a high priority for professionals working in hospital they will be a necessary part of any discharge Care Programme Approach (CPA) planning. It is also recognised that such people suffer iatrogenic side-effects of their treatments (Illich, 1977) and are stigmatised and socially excluded as a direct result of their illness (Rogers et al., 1993). We also know that they are perceived as being vulnerable, and that they risk being disempowered in their care by professionals and become dependent upon the mental health system

(Ryan, 1998). Consequently, less tangible risks such as these may be of greater significance to the patient than those of the professional. For example, the risk of being stigmatised after being admitted to a mental health unit for the first time in their life may be the greatest concern of the patient. This is likely to be a difficult challenge for the nursing team to successfully address, particularly when they are concerned with other forms of more tangible risk. However, working with patient-identified risks is a necessary part of building a therapeutic alliance without which patients merely become objectified. This in turn can reinforce reactive or containment strategies for managing risk rather than encouraging proactive engagement and will affect the culture and milieu of the nursing environment.

Risk prediction, risk perceptions and gender

Ongoing risk assessment is a central part of the risk management process. Mental health professionals are building up a vast knowledge of risk factors and protective factors in relation to suicide, self-harm, violence and other risks that can assist in the risk assessment and management processes. However, given the high degree of false negative predictions (predicting that a risk *will not* materialise when it subsequently occurs) with respect to suicide and false positives (predicting that a risk *will* materialise which then does not happen) in relation to violence there is a need to know more about factors that affect those undertaking risk predictions. The holy grail of having tools that accurately predict future risk is probably an unrealistic goal and therefore we are left with significant degrees of subjectivity when undertaking this work. Some factors that impact on the subjectivity associated with risk assessments (for example, our attitudes and prejudices) can be improved through education and awareness of them and through reflection. Factors such as these have been highlighted for some time in the professional literature with respect to our risk perceptions (Special Hospital Services Authority, 1993).

One factor that we are less able to control for and will contribute to the outcome of risk assessments is gender. Of the limited work that has been undertaken in this area we do know that gender is a significant variable with respect to risk perceptions (Ryan, 1998). Irrespective of any other variable, women and men view risks related to mental illness consistently differently, with women perceiving them to be greater than men. This can have a significant effect on risk management, as the outcome of the risk assessment will partly be dictated by the gender of the person undertaking the assessment. If the risk is regarded differently by men and women, this might explain in part why, in the dynamic of a busy acute ward with a range of professionals undertaking both formal and informal risk assessments, predictions of risk can be inaccurate with fatal results.

Users, informal carers and risk management

Within busy acute wards there can be times when it is very difficult to engage in patient-initiated care that avoids the patient becoming the object of care rather than a collaborator or partner. There is emerging evidence that mental health service users and their close family and friends often have well-developed risk management strategies, even if they do not have the risk language of mental health professionals with which to describe what they do (Ryan, 2000). Admission to an in-patient ward can provide an opportunity to educate patients and families about risk management strategies they can adopt and also build on existing skills they might have already developed.

Managing the risk of self-harm and suicide

People with mental health problems are at much greater risk of harming themselves than of harming others (DoH, 2001) and in comparison with the general population this risk is very significant. In a meta-analysis of existing evidence, Harris and Rice (1997) demonstrated that virtually all mental disorders have an increased risk of suicide with the exception of mental retardation and dementia, while severe mental illness increases risk by as much as 10 times (Allebeck and Allgulander, 1990). Misuse of both drugs and alcohol is strongly associated with suicidal behaviour, with Miles (1977) estimating that 15% of alcohol misusers ultimately kill themselves. Indeed, most of the recent rise in young male suicide is related to higher levels of substance misuse (Needleman and Farrell, 1997). Non-fatal self-harm, the strongest single indicator of future suicide (Williams, 1997), is also known to occur more frequently among those with mental health problems.

Suicide prevention is a major government priority in the United Kingdom (DoH, 1998, 1999a). Among suicides in England and Wales, no fewer than 16% are psychiatric in-patients (DoH, 2001). Clearly, the management of the risk of both self-harm and completed suicide must be a high priority for all mental health staff.

Care versus control

Despite the increased risk of self-harm to in-patients, a merely custodial approach, aiming at prevention at any cost, is not appropriate. Morgan (1979) has documented cases of what he calls 'malignant alienation', whereby a number of his own in-patients, and 55% of a further series, appeared to have killed themselves following a progressive deterioration in their relationships with others, including ward staff. It is likely that one reason for these relationship problems is 'counter-transference', whereby negative attitudes of unconscious malice or aversion are communicated to the patient by staff who are responding to feelings of anxiety or helplessness which the patient has awakened in them (Watts and Morgan, 1994). Moreover, the state of mind of a suicidal person is often best understood as one of hopelessness (Beck et al., 1985). It is essential for staff to be able to respond to the emotional vulnerability of those at risk with an empathic, realisitic but positive approach.

The challenge for in-patient suicide prevention and risk management, then, is to seek a dynamic balance of control with care. If the balance is tipped too much towards control, low self-esteem and low morale may be exacerbated due to communication of distrust, infantilisation and denial of personal rights. If care is emphasised at the expense of appropriate vigilance, however, the results may be tragic.

Steps in managing risk of harm to self

Attitudes

Given the importance of positive attitudes in the care of those at risk, all care staff, whether qualified or unqualified, should receive appropriate training and supervision to promote an understanding of the issues which may lead patients to harm themselves. The national recommendation is that such training should be undertaken at least every three years (DoH, 2001).

It also follows that a consistent, ongoing therapeutic relationship or alliance should be the foundation of any risk management plan. Given the centrality of interpersonal vulnerability in self-harming behaviour, the development of a relationship with a named nurse or other keyworker may itself be therapeutic, while the keyworker who has developed an alliance will be in the ideal position to plan and monitor care across different shifts and groups of staff. Given the nature of mental health problems, developing such a relationship may be a challenge, but it is important to at least achieve some initial degree of rapport if the patient is to be encouraged to communicate, and an accurate assessment of risk

Table 7.1 Factors associated with an increased risk of suicide (adapted from Zametkin et al., 2001)

The following factors are strongly associated with suicide attempts.

- A previous history of a suicide attempt
- A major depressive disorder
- A substance abuse disorder
- Being male (males tend to use more violent methods)
- Living alone
- A history of physical or sexual abuse

In addition, the following may precipitate a suicide attempt.

- Recent dramatic personality change
- Psychosocial stressor
- Talking about death or dying
- Availability of method of suicide
- Altered mental state (agitated, suffering from auditory hallucinations, delusions, intoxication or, following a very troubled episode, suddenly becoming calm)

is to be made. By using active listening skills, the keyworker is able to obtain important information from the patient about self-harming ideation, which the patient would otherwise find difficult to express to a stranger due to guilt and fear. Such rapport thus encourages the gradual development of a therapeutic relationship, helping to prevent destructive malignant alienation.

Assessment

Given the fact that all people with mental health problems are at increased risk of self-harming, all patients must be screened for such risk as part of the overall assessment on admission to in-patient care, preferably using an evidence-based screening instrument (SNMAC, 1999). Unfortunately, standardised risk assessment for suicidal intent is not in widespread use within the United Kingdom, an issue the SNMAC advised should be addressed. However, specific risk factors to include in an assessment are listed in Table 7.1.

Information should be obtained from the client and also, where possible, families, carers and the referrer. Inclusion of additional sources is important as the patient may well be reluctant to divulge suicidal intent. The findings of the assessments should be discussed with the ward team and a level of observation should be set and communicated to the whole of the multidisciplinary team.

The level of risk must be re-assessed formally, at set intervals, and informally, by staff observing and sharing their views of the patient's progress. It has recently been found that in no fewer than 85% of suicides by mental health patients, risk was assessed as being low or absent (DoH, 2001). This is testimony to the challenge presented by risk assessment, which is certainly not an exact science, but it also underlines that in some cases the classic phenomenon of 'false improvement' may have occurred, with patients appearing to have improved in mood, leading to relaxation of vigilance by staff. In other cases, the risk level fluctuates from day to day, even hour to hour, while in still others impulsivity, perhaps due to mental illness or substance misuse, may lead to a sudden, spontaneous suicide.

Care planning

The Care Programme Approach (CPA) (DoH, 1990; revised 2000a) was developed in response to major incidents of harm which illustrated the need for systematic care planning by multidisciplinary teams and agencies, coordinated by a consistent keyworker and seeking to actively involve the patient and relatives and carers. Effective use of the CPA with patients assessed as at-risk is a key aspect of risk management, ensuring that an individual member of staff, such as a named nurse in a ward setting, maintains an overview of the care process, that the expertise of different clinicians is employed, that communication about risk is optimised, and that the care plan is implemented and reviewed appropriately. In addition, the crucial post-discharge period, when the patient is at most risk of self-harm (DoH, 2001), can be prepared for; for example, by ensuring the 'in reach' of community staff before the patient returns home.

Clinical interventions

An individualised care plan should be formulated to take account of the patient's specific needs. Self-harming behaviour should be seen as a symptom of other mental health problems rather than a problem in itself, and the reasons for the behaviour should be sought and addressed. Therefore, any underlying depression should be treated with appropriate and effectively monitored medication and, in some cases, electro-convulsive therapy. This should be followed with specific interventions as part of a treatment package directed at addressing risk triggers. These would include the use of problem-solving therapy, cognitive behavioural therapy, supportive counselling, and assistance with practical issues such as finance, housing or relationships.

Observation

Despite the inconsistencies between mental health trusts reported by the SNMAC (1999) regarding definitions of observation, constant observation has always been a key part of in-patient suicide prevention. Constant observation is a problematic activity, however (Duffy, 1995; Bowers et al., 2000), and is unpopular with both staff and patients. Despite its widespread use in the management of suicidal patients, around one-fifth of in-patient suicides were under either constant or intermittent levels of non-routine observation (DoH, 2001). When employed by skilled staff who try to engage the patient rather than to merely passively observe, however, constant observation can offer therapeutic benefits as well as promote physical safety. To this end, staff should receive appropriate skills-based training, be supported and supervised, and should not be asked to observe patients for longer than an hour at a time (Duffy, 1995). Given the potential for harm through premature reduction of observation levels, this must not take place without careful, documented risk assessment and multidisciplinary agreement. For further information on the use of observation with suicidal patients, see Chapter 8 by Julia Jones and Ann Jackson, titled Observation.

Environmental safety

The high suicide rate in prisons is testimony to the fact that there is no such thing as a 'suicide-proof' environment. However, the development of units which offer a therapeutic ambience through the use of single bedrooms and complex layouts, while very justifiable, has meant that the observation of patients at risk has become more difficult than formerly. The main method of suicide by in-patients is by hanging, most commonly from a curtain rail and using a belt as a ligature (DoH, 2001), and services are now required to ensure that shower curtain rails are non-weight-bearing. It is essential that likely ligature points are removed from anywhere accessible to at-risk patients and that regular audits of the clinical environment are carried out to identify potential suicide hazards such as easily breakable windows.

Self-injury

Self-injuring behaviour which is not intended to have fatal consequences is also seen in in-patient settings. The most common is self-cutting, although people also engage in such behaviours as burning, banging parts of the body or scraping the skin. Self-injury is often associated with personality problems, and often develops as a way of coping with intense negative feelings such as guilt, shame, emptiness or anger (Babiker and Arnold, 1997). Self-injury can arouse negative feelings in staff, and it is essential that they be provided with the opportunity to discuss their feelings in clinical supervision, that they be helped to understand the behaviour through training (preferably with input from users who self-injure), and that appropriate local policies be developed to ensure a consistent and supportive therapeutic approach. Available evidence from people who self-injure suggests that they rarely find simply being made to stop the behaviour without alternatives helpful (Babiker and Arnold, 1997). The most effective methods of managing the risks involved in self-injury involve addressing the underlying causes, promoting the person's health and safety and maintaining a positive and empathetic attitude.

Managing the risk of harm to others

Violence risk assessment

Throughout history most societies have assumed a link between mental disorder and violence to others (Monahan and Steadman, 1994). Although the majority of users of mental health services are not violent, it is clear that a small yet significant minority are violent in in-patient settings and the community (Hiday, 1997). In recent times, particularly following the murder of Jonathon Zito by Christopher Clunis in 1992, there has been increasing concern in the United Kingdom over law and order, specifically the risk of violence, and these issues are now high on the political agenda. Several incidents have received considerable media attention and left a strong impression of the potential dangerousness to the public of individuals with various forms of mental disorder (Ryan, 2000). There is increasing suspicion that the professionals and various institutions which are expected to manage risk in day-to-day life have not performed adequately, reinforced by subsequent official inquiries, some of which reveal serious shortcomings both in the clinical management and supervision of these individuals, and failures in liaison and cooperation between agencies (Reed, 1997). These perceived failures can be linked in the minds of the public with the perception of inadequate service provision – for example, secure in-patient beds in the case of psychiatric services – and with the growing concern that the public are not adequately protected from dangerous individuals by current legislation (DoH, 1999b). Regardless of whether people with mental disorder are more likely to be violent than the non-mentally disordered, it is evident that there are a significant minority of mental health service users who pose a risk to others. This is reinforced by the finding that nurses are the occupational group most at risk of violence (Gallagher, 1999) and staff working in NHS Mental Health Service Trusts are up to eight times more likely to be assaulted than staff working in non-Mental Health Trusts (HSA, 1999: 8).

As clinical decisions on risk are made at all stages of the clinical care process and prioritising treatment need and predicting subsequent outcome of any therapeutic approach will rely heavily upon assessing the level of risk (DoH, 2000b), it is important that mental health service providers have a clear structured approach to violence risk assessment.

Role of mental health nurses in violence risk assessment and management

Risk assessment is an inexact science. Ultimately the decision on the level of risk is based on clinical judgement. Ideally, in practice, decisions on risk should be made by a multidisciplinary team involving all the clinicians involved in the care, treatment and management of the individual being assessed. Mental health nurses play a pivotal role in the assessment and management of risk.

Within in-patient settings mental health nurses are a major source of clinical information which needs to be considered by the clinical team when assessing risks. Mental health nurses are able to observe patients for 24 hours each day and have greater opportunities than other professionals to develop relationships with patients and their family/carers (Allen, 1997). Mental health nurses are constantly making decisions based on the level risk to and/or from service users in these environments; for example, managing crises as they arise, controlling freedom of movement within and outside the mental health facility and maintaining safe levels of supervision and observation. This unique position makes the role of the mental health nurse crucial in the process of assessing and managing violence risk.

In the community, mental health nurses may have a more autonomous role in assessing and managing violence risk. This is especially true if the mental health nurse is identified as the Care Coordinator in accordance with the requirements of the Care Programme Approach (DoH, 1990, 2000a). In fact, mental health nurses are the discipline most likely to take this role (Boyd et al., 1996). Mental health nurses are also involved in the screening of patients in GP referrals, Accident and Emergency and Mentally Disordered Offender court diversion schemes (RCN, 1997). These relatively new roles have significant implications for mental health nurses as they identify, assess and manage risk, not least because their individual legal accountability is increased (Gupta, 1995) and their professional judgement will inevitably be subjected to closer scrutiny, particularly should things go wrong.

Clearly then, the knowledge, skills and experience that mental health nurses possess are crucial to clinical interventions involved in the process of assessing and managing risk.

Risk factors for violence

The factors that provide information about who in a given population is going to be violent have been termed *risk factors*, which are measurable factors that correlate with and precede the outcome of interest (Kraemer et al., 1997), in this case violence. Increasing knowledge of what factors best predict challenging/aggressive behaviour could help mental health nurses to (1) recognise factors predictive/protective of violent and aggressive behaviour; (2) identify targets for intervention and (3) equip them with knowledge and skills to reduce risk to the service user, staff and the public. This should also highlight training needs and areas where improved approaches to care, treatment and management are required as, until clinicians are better informed of the factors associated with violent behaviour, there is little chance of improving the accuracy of risk assessments (Monahan and Steadman, 1994).

There are many studies that have attempted to identify which factors are most closely associated with an increased risk of violence from people with mental disorder. However, the field has been blighted by a number of problems and it is recognised that research in this area is flawed with methodological shortcomings with little consistency in the research approaches (Monahan, 1984). Despite the importance of the subject area there are few consistent studies which investigate fully the heterogeneous nature of violent behaviour in mental health services. However, a number of large multi-factorial studies have explored risk factors for in-patient violence (e.g., Crichton, 1995; Royal College of Psychiatrists, 1998; Almvik et al., 1999); community violence (e.g. Klassen and O'Connor, 1988; Swanson et al., 1990; Monahan et al., 2000); and differences between the mentally disordered and non-mentally disordered in terms of which risk factors predict violence (Bonta et al., 1998). The literature is far from consistent in concluding the most valid risk factors for violence. However, there is evidence that a number of characteristics relating to past history, current functioning, protective influences and the individual's context/environment need to be taken into account when assessing violence risk. These factors, derived from previous research, are summarised in Table 7.2. Consideration of some or all these factors should make the risk assessment process more systematic and transparent, while improving

Table 7.2   Risk and protective factors

Historical	Current presentation		Contextual	Protective
A history of violence (recency, frequency, severity, pattern)

Recent verbal threats

Violent lifestyle and background

Victim of childhood physical and sexual abuse | Alcohol or other substance misuse

Involuntary status

Poor collaboration with suggested treatment and management

Antisocial, explosive or impulsive personality traits | Fear, especially perceived threat from others and fear of imminent attack

Delusions focused on a particular identified person

Command hallucinations to harm others; particularly if perceived as omnipotent

Specific preoccupation with violence

Agitation, anger, excitement, overt hostility or suspiciousness | Safety of environment

Extent of social support

Immediate availability of a weapon

Relationship and proximity to potential victim | Responsive/ compliant with treatment

Good insight

Amotivational

Physical disability

Good rapport with staff

Good social networks

No interest in or knowledge of weapons or the means of violence

Fear of own potential for violence |

risk communication between clinicians as part of a multidisciplinary approach.

The multidisciplinary approach to risk assessment and management

The stages of clinical risk assessment and management may be conceptualised as an ongoing process. This has been described as a *Risk Management Cycle* (Doyle, 1998) and is usually implicit to the provision of good-quality health care and integrated into the Care Programme Approach. The basis of any assessment relies on the accumulation of reliable information and consideration of risk factors. Doyle (1996) found that community mental health nurses used a variety of sources to assess the risk of violence from patients. Those used included interviews, observation, record reviews, liaison with others (clinicians, other agencies, family, significant others), via the therapeutic relationship, physical examinations and intuition. Psychometric tests and rating scales based on actuarial or 'objective' information are also increasingly used to assess risk (e.g., HCR-20: see Webster et al., 1995). These can prove very useful and efficient although they should only be used by people trained in their use and/or under supervision by somebody who is trained in their use (e.g., clinical psychologist, clinical nurse specialist).

The debate as to whether the clinical, 'subjective', or actuarial, 'objective', approach is most relevant to clinical practice is complex. The reality of clinical practice is that tests and scales can help to inform clinical judgement, not replace it as ultimately people make decisions, not tests. There is evidence to suggest that a combination of the clinical and actuarial approach is warranted to structure clinicians' risk judgements, as this may be superior to unaided clinical judgement (McNiel and Binder, 1994; Borum, 1996; Douglas et al., 1999). The *Structured Clinical Judgement Approach*, as described by Hart (1998), attempts to bridge the gap between the scientific (actuarial) approach and the clinical practice of risk assessment. This approach emphasises the need to take account of past history, objective measures, current presentation, context/environment and protective factors, and recognises the reality that the process of clinical risk assessment is a dynamic and continuous process which is mediated by changing conditions (see Dolan and Doyle, 2000; Doyle, 2000).

Ultimately the method used by the mental health nurse to elicit information and assess risk will depend upon the circumstances where the assessment is being carried out, interdisciplinary arrangements, the time constraints involved and the wishes of the person being assessed.

Managing violence risk

The management of risk to others encompasses clinical, health and safety, and public protection (political) issues has to be balanced with the rights of the individual. Indeed, this forms one of the most vociferous debates concerning the radical changes introduced in the proposed reforms to the Mental Health Act (DoH, 2000b) where individuals suffering from a dangerous severe personality disorder who are *considered to be a risk* to others can be admitted for compulsory treatment. Effective risk assessment should therefore be part of risk management, and vice versa, and as behaviour likely to cause harm to others may be symptomatic of many disorders, it is unlikely to be susceptible to any single intervention. Closely examining the factors which have contributed to past violent behaviour should prove fruitful in identifying targets for treatment which may reduce risk. For example, poor anger control – anger management; substance abuse – drug/alcohol therapy; persecutory delusions – cognitive and pharmacological interventions. In summarising the approaches to managing violence risk, Harris and Rice (1997) distinguish between several types of risk management intervention which take account of both security and therapeutic interventions. These include interventions that are as follows.

- **Static** – involves preventing harm via such things as video monitoring, seclusion and locked doors.
- **Dynamic** – aims to prevent harm using control and restraint techniques and electronic tagging as required.
- **Situational** – attempts to restrict access to the means of violence or potential victims; e.g., a paedophile having restricted contact with children.
- **Pharmacological** – involves using medication to alleviate symptoms or reduce arousal.
- **Interpersonal** – mainly by talking using calming and de-escalation techniques and rapport building with a view to developing a therapeutic relationship.
- **Self-control** – helping the service user by psychotherapeutic, psychosocial or pharmacological means to control behaviour.

In clinical practice mental health nurses need to draw upon knowledge, skills and experience from a number of different areas. Broadly speaking, current mental health nursing practice involves applying a bio-psychosocial model. Recently, in parallel with the advances in pharmacological interventions for people with serious mental illness, there has been an increasing emphasis on equipping mental health nurses with the knowledge and skills to carry out psychosocial interventions, largely as a result of the development and implementation of the *Thorn Initiative* training programme (Lancashire et al., 1997). The core modules of the Thorn programme are assertive community treatment, psychological interventions (including cognitive behavioural approaches to delusions and hallucinations), and family interventions. Key elements of the courses include the use of objective assessments and adherence to the principles of evaluation, using simple, reliable measures of change (Gournay, 2000). Up until recently the main focus of training for PSI and the implementation of the interventions has been confined to community settings, yet it is now recognised that mental health nurses working in in-patient settings have been starved of skills and require new training initiatives (SNMAC, 1999). Recent reports have stated that all service users with serious mental illness should have access to psychosocial interventions as a standard part of care (Duggen, 1997; SNMAC, 1999) and evidence suggests that psychosocial interventions may provide lasting benefits by reducing distress associated with positive symptoms, reducing relapse rates and reducing the length of hospital stays, thus improving the overall functioning of service users with severe mental illness and by decreasing the distress of their families (Drury et al., 1996; Lancashire et al., 1997; Wykes et al., 1998).

In relation to the management of violence risk, psychosocial interventions should consequently be an essential part of the practice of clinicians

Table 7.3   Psychosocial interventions for violent behaviour

- Coping strategy enhancement – coping with distress resulting from hallucinations and delusions
- Belief modification – modifying delusions and beliefs about voices
- Case management – assertive outreach, contingency planning, early intervention, relapse prevention, therapeutic alliance
- Family interventions – increasing patient activity and decreasing contact with family, stress management, problem solving
- Anger management – self-monitoring, relaxation, cognitive restructuring
- Medication management – assessment and management of side-effects, self-medication strategies
- Motivational interviewing – encouraging hope and motivation
- Problem-solving approaches – systematic approach to solving problems and dilemmas

working with service users with challenging and aggressive behaviours. The vast majority of service users who are in secure settings have serious mental illness and residual distressing positive symptoms (Ewers and Doyle, 2001). As there is often a link between violent disturbed behaviour and symptoms, any interventions which could increase the service users' self-management should play an integral part of risk assessment and management. New training programmes have been developed for mental health nurses working with forensic populations applying the principles of psychosocial interventions (Gournay, 2000). Psychosocial interventions, and in particular formulation-based cognitive behavioural interventions (Table 7.3), are seen by many as the psychological treatment of choice when working with violent and forensic populations (McGuire, 1995; Novaco et al., 1997; Thomson, 2000; Wong and Gordon, 2000) although further rigorous treatment trials are required in this area.

Although people suffering from mental illnesses contribute little to overall violence in society there is still a significant minority of mental health service users who pose a risk to others, usually to those who work or live with them. Therefore, there is a need for mental health nurses to assess violence risk to try and distinguish between which service users will be violent in in-patient and community settings, and to identify what interventions are required to prevent violence and to minimise the risk to the service user and others. A minimum basic framework for assessing the risk of violence and aggression should include attempts to obtain a history, the use of an objective measure integrated with the assessment of their current presentation, a consideration of the context and identification of protective factors. This approach should assist the mental health nurse in reaching an informed judgement that will result in defensible decision-making.

Conclusion

Competent risk assessment, communication and management within an acute mental health ward can be one of the most difficult challenges any nurse can be asked to fulfil, irrespective of their experience. The concept of risk is currently quite limited within the mental health field and largely has been associated with preventing unwanted high consequence/low frequency events, in particular serious violence and suicide. It is not possible to have acute wards that are 'risk-free'. To attempt this would be likely to decrease the personal freedom of patients further than is currently the case in such environments. There is also no guarantee that achieving a risk-free state would necessarily improve the quality of care or the outcomes from that care as it would be likely to be particularly custodial.

However, there are considerable contributions to the effective and proactive management of risk and that can be achieved to minimise risks such as suicide, self-harm and violence; for example, through knowledge of specific factors likely to increase such risks or protect against them. In addition, recognition that risk is not purely a one-dimensional and negative concept also opens up thinking to explore other outcomes from situations than those that are simply unwanted. Presumably, if an unwanted event does not occur then a desired one does. Reflection on this issue can be particularly significant in the context of rehabilitation and user empowerment. From such a position it therefore becomes possible to manage *towards* desired outcomes and not simply manage *away* unwanted outcomes. It can also encourage support of service users, and their informal carers, to manage risks that they face and pose in ways that establish a user-focused culture in the ward environment whilst also helping to develop skills that will be useful once the user has been discharged from hospital. It is also possible from this position to see that user- and carer-defined risks might be different to those identified by professionals and that working with users as partners is likely to ensure skills development in both the user and the nurse.

Finally, there are a number of issues raised in this chapter that relate to current best practice in relation to risk management, such as knowledge of what patient- or process-related issues might increase or decrease a risk. In addition, there are several other pointers for where future practice development might focus. In particular there is considerable scope for examining aspects of the risk manager (who might be a mental health professional but just as easily be the patient or their informal carer) that might contribute to risk assessment, communication and management decisions.

References

Alberg, C., Hatfield, B. and Huxley, P. (1996) *Learning Materials on Mental Health Risk Assessment*. Manchester: Manchester University Press.

Allebeck, P. and Allgulander, C. (1990) 'Suicide among young men: psychiatric illness, deviant behaviour and substance abuse', *Acta Psychiatrica Scandinavica*, 81: 565–70.

Allen, J. (1997) 'Assessing and managing risk of violence in the mentally disordered', *Journal of Psychiatric and Mental Health Nursing*, 4: 369–78.

Almvik, R., Woods, P. and Rasmussen, K. (1999) 'The Broset Violence Checklist: sensitivity, specificity and interrater reliability', *Journal of Interpersonal Violence*, 15 (12): 1284–96.

Babiker, G. and Arnold, L. (1997) *The Language of Injury: Comprehending Self-mutilation*. Leicester: British Psychological Society.

Beck, A.T., Steer, R.A., Kovacs, M. and Garrison, B. (1985) 'Hopelessness and eventual suicide. A ten year prospective study of patients hospitalised with suicidal ideation', *American Journal of Psychiatry*, 145: 559–63.

Bines, W. (1994) *The Health of Single Homeless People – Discussion Paper 9*. York: Centre for Housing Policy, University of York.

Bonta, J., Law, M. and Hanson, K. (1998) 'The prediction of criminal and violent recidivism among mentally disordered offenders: a meta-analysis', *Psychological Bulletin*, 123 (2): 123–42.

Borum, R. (1996) 'Improving the clinical practice of violence risk assessment', *American Psychologist*, 51 (9): 945–56.

Bowers, L., Gournay, K. and Duffy, D. (2000) 'Suicide and self-harm in in-patient psychiatric units: a national survey of observation policies', *Journal of Advanced Nursing*, 32: 437–44.

Boyd, W., Simms, A. and Brooker, A. (1996) *Boyd Report: Report of the Confidential Inquiry into Homicides and Suicides by Mentally Ill People*. London: Royal College of Psychiatrists.

Crichton, J. (1995) 'A review of psychiatric inpatient violence', in J. Crichton (ed.), *Psychiatric Patient Violence: Risk and Response*. London: Duckworth.

Crisis (1999) *Out of Sight, Out of Mind: The Experiences of Homeless Women*. London: Crisis.

Department of Health (1990) *The Care Programme Approach for People with a Mental Illness Referred to the Special Psychiatric Services*. London: The Stationery Office.

Department of Health (1998) *Saving Lives: Our Healthier Nation*. London: The Stationery Office.

Department of Health (1999a) *National Service Framework for Mental Health: Modern Standards and Service Models*. London: The Stationery Office.

Department of Health (1999b) *Report of the Expert Committee: Review of the Mental Health Act 1983*. London: The Stationery Office.

Department of Health (2000a) *Effective Care Coordination in Mental Health Services: Modernising the Care Programme Approach – A Policy Booklet*. London: The Stationery Office.

Department of Health (2000b) *Reforming the Mental Health Act* (http://www.doh.gov.uk/mentalhealth/whitepaper2000.htm).

Department of Health (2001) *Safety First: Five Year Report of the National Inquiry into Suicide and Homicide by People with Mental Illness*. London: The Stationery Office.

Dolan, M. and Doyle, M. (2000) 'Violence risk prediction: clinical and actuarial measures and the role of the psychopathy checklist', *British Journal of Psychiatry*, 177: 303–11.

Douglas, K., Cox, D. and Webster, C. (1999) 'Violence risk assessment: science and practice', *Legal and Criminological Psychology*, 4: 184–94.

Doyle, M. (1996) 'Assessing risk of violence from clients', *Mental Health Nursing*, 16 (3): 20–3.

Doyle, M. (1998) 'Clinical risk assessment for mental health nurses', *Nursing Times*, 94 (17): 47–49.

Doyle, M. (2000) 'Risk assessment and management', in C. Chaloner and M. Coffey (eds), *Forensic Mental Health Nursing: Current Approaches*. London: Blackwell Science.

Drury, V., Birchwood, M. and Cochrane, R. (1996) 'Cognitive therapy and recovery from acute psychosis: a controlled trial. II. Impact on recovery time', *British Journal of Psychiatry*, 169: 602–7.

Duffy, D. (1995) 'Out of the shadows: a study of the special observation of psychiatric in-patients', *Journal of Advanced Nursing*, 21: 944–50.

Duggen, M. (1997) *Pulling Together: Future Roles and Training for Mental Health Staff.* London: Sainsbury Centre for Mental Health.

Ewers, P. and Doyle, M. (2001) 'The implementation of psychosocial interventions in a forensic mental health service'. Conference Paper Presentation at Creating Seamless Services in Forensic Psychiatry, University of Central Lancashire, 5 June.

Gallagher, J. (1999) *Violent Times: TUC Report on Preventing Violence at Work.* London: Trade Union Congress Health and Safety Unit.

Gournay, K. (2000) 'Role of the community psychiatric nurse in the management of schizophrenia', *Advances in Psychiatric Treatment*, 6: 243–51.

Gupta, N. (1995) 'Keyworkers and the Care Programme Approach. The role and responsibilities of community workers', *Psychiatric Care*, 1: 239–42.

Harris, G. and Rice, M. (1997) 'Risk appraisal and management of violent behaviour', *Psychiatric Services*, 48 (9): 1168–76.

Hart, S.D. (1998) 'The role of psychopathy in assessing risk for violence: conceptual and methodological issues', *Legal and Criminological Psychology*, 3: 121–37.

Hiday, V. (1997) 'Understanding the connection between mental illness and violence', *International Journal of Law and Psychiatry*, 20 (4): 399–417.

Housing Service Agency (HSA) (1999) *The Outreach Directory Annual Statistics 1998–1999*. London: Housing Service Agency.

Illich, I. (1977) *Limits to Medicine, Medical Nemesis: The Expropriation of Health.* Harmondsworth: Penguin.

Klassen, D. and O'Connor, W. (1988) 'Crime, inpatient admissions and violence among male mental patients', *International Journal of Law and Psychiatry*, 11: 305–12.

Kraemer, H., Kazdin, A., Offord, D., Kesler, R., Jensen, P. and Kupfer, D. (1997) 'Coming to terms with the terms of risk', *Archives of General Psychiatry*, 54: 337–43.

Labour Force Survey 1997/8 (1998) 'Unemployment and activity rates for people of working age'. Background paper for Welfare to Work Seminar, Department for Education and Employment, London.

Lancashire, S., Haddock, G., Tarrier, N., Butterworth, T. and Baguley, I. (1997) 'Training community psychiatric nurses in psychosocial interventions in serious mental illness: the Thorn Nurse Initiative', *The Clinician*, 12: 45–8.

McGuire, J. (1995) *What Works: Reducing Reoffending. Guidelines from Research and Practice*. Chichester: Wiley.

McNiel, D.E. and Binder, R.L. (1994) 'Screening for risk of inpatient violence', *Law and Human Behavior*, 18: 579–86.

Miles, C.P. (1977) 'Conditions predisposing to suicide: a review', *Journal of Nervous and Mental Disease*, 164: 231–46.

Monahan, J. (1984) 'The prediction of violent behaviour: toward a second generation of theory and policy', *American Journal of Psychiatry*, 141: 10–15.

Monahan, J. and Steadman, H. (1994) *Violence and Mental Disorder: Developments in Risk Assessments.* Chicago: University of Chicago Press.

Monahan, J., Steadman, H.J., Appelbaum, P.S., Robbins, P.C., Mulvey, E.P., Silver, E., Roth, L.H. and Grisso, T. (2000) 'Developing a clinically useful actuarial tool for assessing violence risk', *British Journal of Psychiatry*, 176: 312–19.

Moore, B. (1996) *Risk Assessment: A Practitioner's Guide to Predicting Harmful Behaviour.* London: Whiting and Birch.

Morgan, H.G. (1979) *Death Wishes? The Understanding and Management of Deliberate Self-Harm.* Chichester: Wiley.

Morgan, S. (1998) *Assessing and Managing Risk: Practitioner's Handbook.* Brighton: Pavilion/Sainsbury Centre for Mental Health.

Needleman, J. and Farrell, M. (1997) 'Suicide and substance misuse', *British Journal of Psychiatry*, 171: 303–4.

Novaco, R. (1997) 'Remediating anger and aggression with violent offenders', *Legal and Criminological Psychology*, 2: 77–88.

Prins, H. (1999) *Will They Do It Again?* London: Routledge.

Reed, J. (1997) 'Risk assessment and clinical risk management: the lessons from recent inquiries', *British Journal of Psychiatry*, 170 (Supplement 32): 4–7.

Rogers, A., Pilgrim, D. and Lacey, R. (1993) *Experiencing Psychiatry. Users' Views of Services.* London: Macmillan.

Royal College of Nursing (RCN) (1997) *Buying Forensic Mental Health Nursing: An RCN Guide for Purchasers.* London: RCN.

Royal College of Psychiatrists (1998) 'Management of imminent violence: clinical practice guidelines to support mental health services', Occasional Paper OP41, Royal College of Psychiatrists, London, March.

Ryan, T. (1998) 'Perceived risks associated with mental illness: beyond homicide and suicide', *Social Science and Medicine*, 46 (2): 287–97.

Ryan, T. (1999) *Managing Crisis and Risk in Mental Health Nursing.* Cheltenham: Nelson Thornes.

Ryan, T. (2000) 'Exploring the risk management strategies of mental health service users', *Health, Risk and Society*, 2 (3): 267–82.

Singleton, N., Meltzer, H., Gatwood, R., Coid, J. and Deasy, D. (1998) *Psychiatric Morbidity among Prisoners in England and Wales: The Report of a Survey carried out in 1997 by Social Survey Division of the Office for National Statistics on behalf of the Department of Health.* London: The Stationery Office.

Special Hospital Services Authority (1993) *Report of the Committee of Inquiry into the Death in Broadmoor Hospital of Orville Blackwood and a Review of the Death of Two Other Afro-Caribbean Patients: 'Big, Black and Dangerous?'.* London: Special Hospital Services Authority.

Standing Nursing and Midwifery Advisory Committee (SNMAC) (1999) *Practice Guidance: Safe and Supportive Observation of Patients at Risk.* London: The Stationery Office.

Swanson, J., Holzer, C., Ganju, V. and Jono, R. (1990) 'Violence and psychiatric disorder in the community: evidence from the Epidemiological Catchment Area Surveys', *Hospital and Community Psychiatry*, 41: 761–70.

Thomson, L.D. (2000) 'Management of schizophrenia in conditions of high security', *Advances in Psychiatric Treatment*, 6: 252–60.

Watts, D. and Morgan, H.G. (1994) 'Malignant alienation', *British Journal of Psychiatry*, 164: 11–15.

Webster, C., Harris, G., Rice, M., Cormier, C. and Quinsey, V. (1995) *The HCR-20 Scheme: The Assessment of Dangerousness and Risk*. Vancouver: Simon Fraser University/British Columbia Forensic Psychiatric Services Commission.

Williams, M. (1997) *Cry of Pain: Understanding Suicide and Self-harm*. Penguin: Harmondsworth.

Wong, S. and Gordon, A. (2000) *Violence Reduction Programme: Phases of Treatment and Content Overview*. Saskatoon, Saskatchewan, Canada: Regional Psychiatric Centre.

Wykes, T., Tarrier, N. and Lewis, S. (1998) *Outcome and Innovation in Psychological Innovation in Schizophrenia*. Chichester: Wiley.

Zametkin, A.J., Alter, M.R., and Yemini, T.B.A. (2001) 'Suicide in teenagers: assessment, management and prevention', *Journal of the American Medical Association*, 286 (24): 3120–5.

EIGHT
Observation

Julia Jones and Ann Jackson

Introduction

A report in *The Guardian* newspaper in September 1999 told the sad story of a talented playwright called Sarah Kane who committed suicide at the age of 28 (Guardian, 1999). She has been hailed as 'the young playwright of her generation' yet her professional success was blighted by a long history of severe depression. In the two years before her death she had been in and out of psychiatric care, and her illness finally resulted in her taking her life. The story is tragic. What is even more tragic is that Sarah Kane took her life when she was in hospital, where she should have been 'safe'. According to *The Guardian* newspaper report, medical staff had recognised her suicidal risk as she had been admitted three days earlier after a suicide attempt from taking an overdose of anti-depressants and sleeping pills. However, the two psychiatrists who assessed Sarah Kane did not communicate to nursing staff that she should be observed closely because of her high risk. A psychiatrist told the coroner's court that he 'took it as read' that she would be 'constantly observed' by nursing staff. The nursing staff therefore had not been 'directly' informed that she required special monitoring. Shortly after 3.30 a.m. on 20 September 1999 a nurse found Sarah Kane hanging from the hook inside the toilet door, hanging by a shoelace. She had not been seen by nursing staff for 90 minutes.

We acknowledge that this is just one tragic case, and our intention is not to sensationalise it or make judgements, as none of us knows the full details of what happened. The purpose of discussing this case is that so many of the things that went wrong in the care of Sarah Kane have been highlighted as being endemic in the care of suicidal patients in acute in-patient care. Key findings from *Safety First, Five-Year Report of the National Confidential Inquiry into Suicide and Homicide by People with Mental Illness* (DoH, 2001) bear a strong resemblance to the circumstances that contributed to the suicide of Sarah Kane. Of particular significance are the following findings from the Inquiry: that approximately one-quarter (24%)

of people who had committed suicide had been in contact with mental health services in the year before their death; 16% of all suicide inquiry cases in England and Wales (12% in Scotland and 10% in Northern Ireland) were psychiatric in-patients; in-patient suicides account for 4% of all suicides in the UK population; in-patient suicides, particularly those occurring on the ward, were most likely to be by hanging; around one-quarter of in-patient suicides died during the first week of admission. Regarding observation specifically, around one-fifth of in-patient suicides occurred when patients were under non-routine observation (constant and intermittent), and many in-patient suicides were associated with reported difficulties in observing patients because of ward design (24%) and where wards had a shortage of nurses (25%) (Appleby et al., 1999; DoH, 2001).

The main circumstance that is not relevant to the case of Sarah Kane is that she was not being observed closely by nursing staff at the time of her death. But even when psychiatric in-patients are placed on observation, the Confidential Inquiry Report (DoH, 2001) demonstrates that this nursing intervention is not always effective in keeping people safe from harm. Concerns about the standards of care provided in in-patient settings, particularly regarding patients' safety, stimulated the report on which this book is based – *Mental Health Nursing: Addressing Acute Concerns* (DoH, 1999a) – which was produced by the Standing Nursing and Midwifery Advisory Committee (SNMAC). The concern regarding the practice of observation prompted a focus of the report to review policies and procedures for observation at a national level (England and Wales) and to produce practice guidance on *Safe and Supportive Observation of Patients at Risk* (Department of Health, 1999b). This guidance, known commonly as the 'SNMAC Practice Guidance on Observation', is intended to be a template for local services to use in developing protocols and practice.

This chapter will discuss the policy and practice of observation in acute in-patient psychiatric settings for adults, drawing upon the *Addressing Acute Concerns* report, highlighting the existing research and practice 'evidence'[1] for the safe and supportive observation of patients[2] at risk. The chapter will also discuss the research literature that has explored nurses' and patients' experiences and views of observation. The aim of the chapter therefore is to provide current research and practice 'evidence' regarding how observation should be carried out in an effective and supportive way,

---

[1]Our use of the term 'evidence' denotes our current philosophical stance. Evidence coming from practice is given equal importance within the hierarchy of valid evidence. We have endeavoured to make such 'evidence' distinct from research findings (as only one form of evidence).

[2]We use the term 'patient' consciously within this chapter. Whilst we would otherwise pursue a less paternalistic term, and are aware of the ongoing and often irreconcilable debates around language, we believe that in relation to this specific area of practice, the term 'patient' more realistically and authentically describes the role of the patient receiving professional care.

whilst maintaining patients' safety, dignity, autonomy and identity as a 'person' rather than simply a 'patient'.

Purpose of observation

The observation of patients at risk is a key component of psychiatric in-patient nursing care. It is a commonly used nursing intervention for patients 'at-risk', and involves the allocation of one nurse (or sometimes two) to one patient for a prescribed length of time in order to provide intensive nursing care. The main purpose of conducting observation is to keep people safe when they are acutely mentally ill and disturbed, particularly patients who are assessed to be at-risk of harming themselves or others, or at-risk of being harmed or exploited by others. Observation is typically used for patients who are suicidal or actively interested in harming themselves, patients who are aggressive and who pose a danger to staff or other patients, vulnerable patients, those who are prone to abscond, and those patients who are sexually disinhibited (Bowers et al., 2000; Bowers and Park, 2001). Three main types of patients are most likely to be observed intensively by nurses: young male schizophrenia sufferers who are deemed to be suicidal or who have behavioural problems; older depressed and suicidal female patients; and patients suffering from a personality disorder (Phillips et al., 1977; Childs et al., 1994).

According to the SNMAC practice guidance on the *Safe and Supportive Observation of Patients at Risk* (Department of Health, 1999b), observation (p. 2) is defined as

> regarding the patient attentively while minimising the extent to which they feel that they are under surveillance.

The challenge for nurses who conduct observation is to maintain the safety of 'high-risk' patients, whilst maintaining their dignity, privacy and autonomy. For nurses, observing a patient who is deeply distressed and potentially suicidal or aggressive is one of the most difficult and demanding roles to undertake. This is recognised by the SNMAC practice guidance for observation (Department of Health, 1999b), with the guidance highlighting the inherent tension of the nursing observation procedure. On page 2, the guidance states that

> whereas most nursing interventions are intended to help patients achieve their own goals, observation is deliberately designed to frustrate patients' aims.

Thus 'keeping someone safe' may in reality mean having to stop a patient from doing something they are intent on doing; for example: leaving the unit; attempting to harm themselves in some way; or behaving aggressively towards others. For nurses, having to act in such a way can appear custodial and dehumanising to patients, and also go against the humanistic ideals of many mental health nurses who strive to maintain a therapeutic relationship with patients (Duffy, 1995). These practice dilemmas faced by nurses when conducting observation are addressed in greater detail later in this chapter.

Regarding the terminology used to describe the procedure of observation, there is no universal term used. Instead the procedure is known by various terms; for example: special, close, maximum, continuous or constant observation, attention or supervision; suicide watch or precaution; 15-minute or intermittent checks; specialling; one-to-one nursing; nursing observation; formal observation (this list is derived from Bowers and Park, 2001, and our own experience from visiting different acute settings). In this chapter, for purposes of consistency, the term 'observation' will be used.

The procedure of observation is generally carried out according to different prescribed 'levels' of observation, which vary in intensity according to the degree of perceived risk. Patients assessed to be at greatest risk of harming themselves or others are nursed on the highest level of observation, with patients never being left alone by nurses, and with the nurse often within 'arm's reach' of the patient. This most intensive form of nursing observation is also known by several different terms; for example: constant observation; maximum observation; level 1 observation; special observation; and specialling. However, the way that these levels are used, and how observation is conducted in general in the UK, varies considerably at the local level, with the use of different terminology, policies and practice.

Policies and procedures

Despite national initiatives to standardise observation policies and procedures, the present situation is that policies are developed and implemented at the local level (i.e., within an individual trust). Little published guidance exists, apart from Ritter's (1989) manual of practice guidance which was a product of her work on observation policy and procedure at the Bethlem and Maudsley Hospitals in London. There also now exists the SNMAC practice guidance document (Department of Health, 1999b), although this only applies to England and Wales. In Scotland there is the Good Practice Statement for *Nursing Observation of Acutely Ill Psychiatric Patients in Hospital* (CRAG/SCOTMEG, 1995), although the most up-to-date information can be found on the CRAG website (www.show.scot.nhs.uk/crag/).

The national picture

Despite the frequent occurrence of this nursing intervention in acute psychiatric settings, for the UK as a whole there are no national standards or guidelines for the practice of observation. As already mentioned, the SNMAC practice guidance for the observation of patients at risk (Department of Health, 1999b) has been produced and is recommended by the Department of Health to act as a template for local services in England and Wales developing their own policies and procedures. However, without any follow-up evaluation of the adoption of this guidance, the impact of this practice guidance is unclear. Anecdotal 'evidence', derived from visiting different trusts and talking to nurses, would suggest that by the beginning of 2002 many trusts in England and Wales had revised their observation policies to incorporate the SNMAC guidance. However, the authors were also aware of local trusts whose local observation policies remain unchanged since the publication of the SNMAC practice guidance in 1999. Thus it seems likely that there is great variation between trusts that have adopted the SNMAC guidance in its entirety, those trusts that have adopted some components of the guidance, and some trusts who have not revised their observation policies at all. At the present time there has been no national audit to explore the extent of implementation of the SNMAC guidance at a national level. Furthermore, as stated by Bowers et al. (2000), evaluation into the efficacy of the observation procedures contained in the SNMAC guidance is also required.

The SNMAC practice guidance was in part the result of a survey commissioned by the Department of Health as part of the Addressing Acute Concerns programme, to investigate how observation was being conducted locally across England and Wales. A sample of 27 psychiatric in-patient providers in England and Wales responded by sending details of their local policies and procedures for observation. The findings of the survey are detailed in Bowers et al. (2000). But to summarise, the survey found that the policies and practice of observation in England and Wales vary considerably. The most prominent findings of the study were the huge variation in terminology and content of different observation policies, and also which staff (qualified or non-qualified, permanent or bank/agency staff) were conducting the procedure. More than 1 in 10 services of the sample had no written observation policy, and 4 in 10 had no clinical recording system of the procedure in place. This survey demonstrated that at the time of the survey, in many localities nursing observation operates according to local tradition rather than upon any evidence of what is clinically effective.

Elsewhere in the UK the picture is similar; i.e., that the policies and practice for observation are variable and non-standardised. In Scotland a written 'good practice statement' regarding nursing observation has been in existence since 1995 (CRAG/SCOTMEG, 1995); it has been adopted in a number of trusts and some local audits have been conducted (see, for example, Porter et al., 1998). However, at a national level there has been no evaluative work conducted to assess the extent of implementation or effectiveness of the guidance (Kettles, 2000). There is no national guidance for the practice of nursing observation available in Northern Ireland. As in the rest of the UK, in Northern Ireland observation policies and procedures remain the domain of individual trusts and hospitals.

The local picture

It is clear that from the work conducted by Bowers et al. (2000) in England and Wales that there is enormous variation in the way that observation is being conducted in different trusts and hospitals. There is also evidence that within individual trusts, the practice of observation may vary. An audit of observation procedures in a Scottish NHS trust showed that not only were there variations in the use of observation between different wards but also between consultant psychiatrists (Porter et al., 1998). Similar variations have been uncovered by other studies; for example, an audit conducted in a single trust in England by Neilson and Brennan (2001) found a variation in the use of different levels of observation across four different wards and in the documentation of the risk factors. Variations of this type have also been found during a study of patients' experience of observation (Jones et al., 2000a, 2000b). During a three-month period, data were obtained from the numbers of patients being observed across five acute in-patient wards in a single NHS trust in England. The use of different levels of observation, and the amount of time that particular patients remained on higher levels of observation, varied considerably across the five wards.

Similar findings are also reported by Bowers and Park (2001). So why is there so much variation in the way that observation is carried out and documented within a single trust or hospital? There is no conclusive evidence to answer this question, although the findings of different research studies do offer possible suggestions. The work of Porter et al. (1998) highlighted that different consultant psychiatrists in a single trust displayed different patterns of usage, with some consultants placing patients on observation for longer time periods than others. This could be put down to 'defensive' practice, although Porter et al. (1998) stated that a consultant with the highest number of hours consulted nursing staff more than many other consultants and was held in esteem by his colleagues. Another possible reason highlighted by Porter et al. (1998) and Neilson and Brennan (2001) is that even when most nurses display good knowledge of the local observation policy and procedure, errors and inconsistencies in documentation are widespread. However, it cannot always be taken for granted that all staff have a good knowledge of the local Trust observation policy, as demonstrated by Midence et al. (1996), who found that nursing staff were often not familiar with their trust's observation procedures. A similar 'lack of knowledge' from staff was uncovered during the observation study conducted by one of the authors (Jones et al., 2000a) when patient respondents commented that some nursing staff, in particular students, bank and agency staff, appeared to have a limited knowledge of the observation procedure.

A further possible reason to explain local variations in the observation procedure could be that where decisions regarding the observation of patients are not multidisciplinary, but made predominantly by medical staff and then conducted by nursing staff, then frequently nurses modify the operational procedure. A study conducted in Canada by Aidroos (1986) found that only 24% of the observations of patients conducted by nurses during a 4-month period (284 different 'units' of observation were directly observed) conformed more or less to the local hospital's policy, with 41% of the observations conducted being totally non-compliant. The main reason for the modification of 'doctors' orders' by nurses offered by Aidroos was that the nurses she studied used their own clinical judgement according to patients' current condition, rather than 'doctors' orders' that were often considered to be 'erroneous, stale or forgotten' (p. 833). In other words, the nurses observed patients solely according to their own professional judgement. Aidroos (1986) in turn questioned the need for doctors to be involved in decision-making about observation, apart from when patients are at a high risk of harm, suggesting that nurses have the adequate skills to make such decisions.

Similar findings to Aidroos (1986) have been suggested by studies conducted elsewhere in the UK. From a study focusing upon the care of suicidal patients by nurses, Duffy (1995) found that despite the official policy for the conduct of observation, nurses would frequently 'modify' the prescribed methods and care plans from medical and other nursing staff if they considered that it was in the patients' interests to do so. Duffy (1995) concluded that such a 'flexible' approach was in part acceptable in that the patients observed in this way came to no harm. However, if a patient does harm themselves in such circumstances, without a formal nursing assessment to support a nurse's action, then this situation can be difficult to reconcile within an official policy.

Some key principles regarding local observation policies and procedures

This section summarises some of the key areas of guidance provided for local observation policies from the SNMAC practice guidance for England and Wales (DoH, 1999b) and the CRAG/SCOTMEG (1995) good-practice statement for Scotland.

All local trusts and hospitals should have a written policy for the safe and supportive observation of patients at-risk. One would think that it is unnecessary to make this statement. However, the survey conducted by Bowers et al. (2000) for the 'Addressing Acute Concerns' report found that three of the 27 trusts surveyed in England and Wales did not have a written policy on observation. Furthermore, policies should be formulated with wide local consultation, involving professionals from all relevant disciplines, patient and carer representatives.

Local policies and procedures for the safe and supportive observation of patients at-risk should not be considered separately from the processes of risk assessment and care planning. The observation of patients 'at-risk' should not be conducted in isolation from a robust risk assessment process, which is multidisciplinary and whenever possible involves patients and their carers/families. A detailed risk assessment should be carried out on all newly admitted patients by the medical and nursing staff who are responsible for admitting the patient. Following this initial assessment, risk must be assessed at regular agreed intervals. Again, this is a fundamental principle that at the present time is not occurring in all localities, as demonstrated by the Bowers et al. (2000) survey which found that 14 of the 27 trusts surveyed did not even have a written risk assessment policy. Similarly, observation should be conducted within a formulated nursing care plan which clearly sets out the therapeutic goals of the admission and the specific nursing interventions to support the patient/client through the acute phase of their illness/distress.

Local policies and procedures for the safe and supportive observation of patients at-risk should be audited and reviewed regularly. It is recommended that local policies for observation should be audited regularly, and the SNMAC practice guidance recommends auditing at six-monthly intervals. The authors also recommend an annual review of the actual policy to accommodate findings from local audits and any published research on observation or national recommendations.

All clinical staff involved in the observation of patients at-risk should be provided with adequate training, supervision and support to equip them with the required knowledge of the local policy and the skills to conduct the procedure. The written policy on observation should be available in all clinical areas and this should form part of the induction and orientation process for all new staff (qualified, unqualified, other clinical staff, bank and agency staff, and students) in a ward or unit. The authors suggest that such training should also be updated at regular intervals, perhaps every 12 months. According to the SNMAC practice guidance, essential components of adequate training include the following: risk assessment; management and engagement of patients at-risk of harming self or others; factors associated with self-harm/harm to others; indications for observation (i.e., indicators of risk); levels of observation; attitudes to observation; therapeutic opportunities in observation; roles and responsibilities of the multidisciplinary team in relation to observation; making the environment safe; recording observation; the use of reviews and audit.

All trusts and hospitals should provide adequate written information about observation for patients and their carers/families. One of the most negative things patients report about observation is not being provided with adequate information regarding what it is, why it is used and what it means in respect to their care while in hospital. It is considered good practice for all in-patient providers to have written information on observation, that is written in a simple and jargon-free language that is easy for non-professionals to understand. There are some excellent information packs that have been developed by some local trusts, in particular those produced in partnership with patients and carers.

The practice of observation

Observation requires qualified, experienced nursing staff to be with the patient at times of great distress and potential danger (to themselves or others). Its purpose is life-saving and is both safe and therapeutic, with the aim of maintaining positive engagement. However, the practice of observation in many places has become diluted and compromised by cultural and structural problems operating within acute areas (Barker and Cutcliffe, 1999; Dodds and Bowles, 2001). Although it is difficult to generalise how observations should be done, indeed there is little researched evidence to make such recommendations, the following are the six key areas that should be considered to maintain a patient-centred focus.

Level of observation

A key area of observation practice is making decisions regarding the intensity of care required for individual patients. The decision to use observation, and which level of intensity is required, should be based upon a multidisciplinary assessment of risk (as discussed previously). The SNMAC practice guidance for England and Wales (DoH, 1999b) recommends the use of four levels of observation; see Table 8.1.

**Table 8.1   Four levels of observation detailed in SNMAC practice
guidance (reproduced with kind permission from the DoH)**

Four levels of observation

In order to facilitate communication, care planning and training, the following classification
in the level of observation is recommended:

Level I. *General observation* is the minimum acceptable level of observation for all
in-patients. The location of all patients should be known to staff, but not all patients need to
be kept within sight. At least once a shift a nurse should sit down and talk with each
patient to assess their mental state. This interview should always include an evaluation
of the patient's mood and behaviours associated with risk and should be recorded in
the notes.

Level II. *Intermittent observation* means that the patient's location must be checked every 15
to 30 minutes (exact times to be specified in the notes). This level is appropriate when
patients are potentially, but not immediately, at risk. Patients with depression, but no immediate plans to harm themselves or others, or patients who have previously been at risk of harm
to self or others, but who are in a process of recovery, require intermittent observation.

Level III. *Within eyesight* is required when the patient could, at any time, make an attempt
to harm themselves or others. The patient should be kept within sight at all times, by day
and night and any tools or instruments that could be used to harm self or others should be
removed. It may be necessary to search the patients and their belongings whilst having
due regard for patients' legal rights.

Level IV. *Within arm's length:* patients at the highest levels of risk of harming themselves
or others, may need to be nursed in close proximity. On rare occasions more than one
nurse may be necessary. Issues of privacy, dignity and consideration of the gender in allo-
cating staff, and the environmental dangers, need to be discussed and incorporated into
the care plan.

The four levels detailed by the SNMAC report are not based upon
'evidence' as such, as they have not been evaluated. They are instead
recommended as guidance to local services in England and Wales, intended
to provide a template for local policies. However, local trusts and hospitals are not required in any legal sense to adopt these levels in their
entirety, and therefore it is likely that there remains great variation in the
terminology and detail of observation levels used in different places.
Partly this may still be due to poor awareness of the report itself, or trusts
only incorporating elements of the SNMAC guidance rather in its entirety.
Second, organisations often need more than recommended guidance to
change practice, which is embedded in the culture of individual wards and
clinical teams.

It is important to note the differences between the guidance issued for
Scotland and the SNMAC guidance for England and Wales. In Scotland,
the CRAG/SCOTMEG (1995) *Good Practice Statement*, which has been
adopted in a number of Scottish trusts (Porter et al., 1998), has just three
levels of observation: *General Observation*; *Constant Observation*; and

Special Observation. As well as the difference in the number of levels of observation recommended, and the terminology used, a further variation between the two practice statements is that the SNMAC guidance recommends the use of intermittent observation, whereas the CRAG/SCOTMEG guidance does not. This difference is a significant one, and represents differences in opinion amongst many mental health practitioners regarding the usefulness of intermittent observation, which involves the regular checking of patients' whereabouts at timed intervals (e.g., every 15 or 30 minutes). Intermittent observation can be seen as being less intense and less intrusive, particularly when the intensity of observation is being reduced.

However, there are a number of negative concerns regarding such 'timed checks'. These focus on the view that the use of intermittent observation is unsafe, because an individual can carry out risk behaviours during the gaps between observations, and that this therefore does not fulfil the purpose of observation. It seems likely that the revised Scottish guidance will continue to not recommend the use of intermittent observation in the revised guidance document. Such concerns are also highlighted in the *Safety First* report (DoH, 2001), which reported that 18% of all in-patient suicides occurred when patients were being observed at intervals of 5–30 minutes. The report states that 'intermittent observations, in particular, are of unproven benefit even when they are carried out properly' (p. 146). The report recommends that patients who are at present placed under intermittent observation should be under continuous one-to-one placement, or that alternative approaches should be adopted such as having areas of the ward being constantly observed or the ward exit. However, it should be noted that the effectiveness of such alternatives are also unproven.

The decision-making process

Both the SNMAC guidance and the CRAG/SCOTMEG good practice statement recommend that, wherever possible, decisions about observation should be made jointly by the multidisciplinary team. Such a decision should be based upon an assessment of risk, using an evidence-based risk assessment tool, a consideration of the patient's history and an interview with the patient and his/her carer or advocate (as requested by the patient). Decisions regarding observation are made at various stages of the procedure: whether or not observation is required; on which level of observation to place a patient; whether to either increase or decrease the intensity of observation; and when to terminate observation. These decisions should also be reviewed regularly. The SNMAC guidance recommends that a patient's observation status should be reviewed by a doctor and the primary nurse or ward sister/charge nurse every day (including weekends). For the most intensive level of observation – within arms' length – then there should be three reviews: two during the day and one during the night shift (DoH, 1999b).

It is highly desirable that all decisions regarding observation should be made jointly by the multidisciplinary team. It is acknowledged, though, that this is not always possible, particularly at weekends and evenings, when often it will be a junior or duty doctor and the ward nursing team who make these decisions. However, it has been demonstrated that the involvement of nurses in such decision-making varies greatly from ward to ward, and hospital to hospital. For example, Childs et al. (1994) found that the use of observation is initiated more often by medical staff on their own than by nurses or as a multidisciplinary team decision. Duffy (1995) reported from his study that it was always medical staff who initiated or terminated observation, although this was often based upon information provided by nursing staff. At the setting where one of the authors was researching observation (Jones et al., 2000a, 2000b), nurses were able to initiate observation and place patients on more intense levels, but were unable to terminate observation or reduce the intensity of observation level without permission from medical staff. Such evidence suggests that despite the rhetoric or multidisciplinary team decision-making, there remains great variation across the UK regarding the role of nurses in making decisions about the observation of patients at risk. This remains the case, despite the fact that nurses carry the major responsibility for conducting the intervention.

Regarding how to make decisions about observation, it is indisputable that this should be based upon an assessment of risk. But, as noted by Bowers and Park, 'risk assessment is an inexact science at the best of times' (2001: 773). The issue of risk assessment is discussed elsewhere in this book, and thus will not be repeated here, but it is worth noting that there is little guidance regarding the decision-making process for observation. The only attention paid to this issue is by Dennis (1997), who interviewed nursing staff about patients who had been observed closely because of the risk of absconding. From this study, Dennis devised two 'decision trees' to help staff consider the options when working with patients at risk of absconding. In particular the decision trees focus on making decisions about whether or not to place a patient on observation, and then when to decrease the intensity of observation.

Finally, it is essential that all decisions are recorded in a patient's clinical notes by a member of the multidisciplinary team. The SNMAC practice guidance states that the records should include the following information:

- current mental state;
- current assessment of risk;

- specific level of observation to be implemented;
- clear directions regarding therapeutic approach; i.e., occupational therapy sessions;
- timing of next review.

It is also specified that the records should include the name of the person conducting the observation, the time they commenced and concluded their period of observation. It is also recommended that a detailed record of the patient's behaviour, mental state and attitude to observation be recorded every 15 minutes.

Such guidance, if implemented, should ensure accurate and clinically useful recording of an individual's care. However, on the evidence of audits, such rigorous record keeping is not always observed. Porter et al. (1998) and Neilson and Brennan (2001) demonstrated substantial inconsistencies in record keeping, with missing or inaccurate information in patients' records regarding their care whilst being observed. Examples included: missing staff names and signatures; lack of information for long periods of time; the times when observations were changed or reduced not clearly documented; alterations to written information, the use of correction fluid; poor information regarding patients' mental state that bore no relevance to the stated risks (such as 'watching TV', 'settled', or 'resting in bed'). Not only does such poor record keeping limit the ability to maintain a continual assessment of patients at risk, it also has legal implications as mental health professionals have a duty of care and are accountable for their actions, decisions and omissions. Thus if a nurse omits to record certain information in a patient's records, or fails to communicate important information, concerns and/or observations to the appropriate team members, then a nurse could be seen to be acting negligently.

Who should observe?

There is considerable debate whether patients at-risk should always be observed by a permanent qualified member of staff, or whether it is acceptable for support workers, students or non-permanent (e.g., agency) staff to conduct this role. In practice, a variety of people perform the 'observer' role, including qualified nurses, agency nurses, nursing and medical students, support workers, family members, friends and volunteers (Bowers and Park, 2001). Observation is often regarded as an unpleasant low-status and low-skill task and frequently delegated to either junior staff, or agency and bank staff who may be unknown to the patient (Barker and Cutcliffe, 1999; Dodds and Bowles, 2001). The reasons for this are complex and debatable, but include: problems of recruitment and retention of qualified and experienced nursing staff in acute in-patient units

(DoH, 1999a, 2001); a reliance on the use of bank and agency staff in many acute in-patient units, particularly in urban areas (Ward et al., 1998); the huge expense of intensive one-to-one observations, estimated by Moore et al. (1995) to absorb up to 20% of the total nursing budget; and that acute in-patient psychiatric wards are increasingly perceived (by staff and patients) as a non-therapeutic environment (SCMH, 1998; DoH, 1999a).

The SNMAC practice guidance adopts a pragmatic position on this issue, stating

it is impossible to stipulate exactly who should carry out this task. (DoH, 1999b: 4)

The fact that observation is described as a 'task' is interesting, although the guidance does also discuss observation in terms of being a 'highly skilled activity'.

Both the SNMAC practice guidance and the SCOT/CRAGMEG good practice statement report that the qualified nurse remains accountable if unqualified nurses or students are allocated the role of observer for patients at risk. The SCOT/CRAGMEG good practice statement cautions on the use of non-qualified nursing staff, stating the need for ensuring that the person delegated this duty must be informed why the patient is being observed and the purpose of the observation. The SNMAC guidance adopts a similar standpoint, stating that it is

undesirable for someone who does not know the ward or the patient to be responsible for observing a patient who is suicidal, vulnerable or violent. (DoH, 1999b: 4)

From the patient's perspective such a situation is also highly undesirable. Patients interviewed by Jones et al. (2000b) stated that being observed by someone they did not know made them feel less safe.

Whether or not patients are observed by nurses they know appears to be connected to organisational factors such as staff shortages, which frequently result in the necessity of employing agency and bank staff to conduct observations. It is acknowledged that nurses struggle with huge bureaucratic demands (Allen, 1998; Higgins et al., 1999), and that the qualified permanent staff have the responsibility to coordinate the shift. However, it is suggested that more attention be given to who actually conducts nursing observation, with a greater emphasis placed upon providing positive therapeutic care by a skilled practitioner, with whom a patient feels comfortable. Even when it is necessary to employ bank and agency staff, who are unknown to patients, it can be argued that one of the key skills of mental health nurses is to be able to establish rapport with people relatively quickly to engage them in a therapeutic relationship.

Involving patients and carers in observation

A guiding value of the *National Service Framework for Mental Health* (DoH, 1999c) is that patients and their carers are involved in the planning and delivery of their care. However, in reality this is not always the case. Much of the research that focuses upon the patient perspective of observation suggests that a major complaint among patients is that they are sometimes not even told that they are being observed. Even when they are told, often it is not explained clearly to them and they rarely feel involved in the decision-making about this component of their care.

Although giving information could be viewed as a procedural matter, with little bearing on the nurse/patient interaction, it can equally be considered an important opportunity to involve patients in their care. This issue yet again highlights the importance of nurse/patient relationships which are open and supportive, and which convey a sense of respect for the patient and their autonomy. It is therefore imperative that every effort is made to involve patients and their carers/friends in the decision-making process, making certain that the procedure and the reasons for its implementation are clearly explained, and ensuring that the observation is conducted in a way that is both supportive and therapeutic.

Gender, ethnicity and culture

The issues of gender, ethnicity and culture remain relatively 'invisible' in the literature on observation. Regarding gender, two quantitative studies show that women are placed on more intensive levels of observation compared to men (Shugar and Rehaluk, 1990; Kettles, 2001), although the reasons for this are not clear. Further exploratory research is required, within the context of the care and safety of women in acute inpatient psychiatric settings, a topic highlighted in reports by the Sainsbury Centre for Mental Health (1997; 1998) and in *Addressing Acute Concerns* (DoH, 1999a). Regarding the practice of observation, we believe that it is important to ask women (and also men) if they prefer an observer of the same or different gender, as far as staffing situations allow. This is particularly important when a nurse needs to accompany a patient to the bathroom. Gender issues regarding observation clearly require greater attention than they currently receive.

In the *National Visit 2* (SCMH, 2000) it was reported that patients from black and minority ethnic communities were often not receiving care that was sensitive to their cultural backgrounds. To our knowledge no research has examined observation from the perspective of ethnicity and culture. It has been demonstrated that within the mental health care system ethnic minority patients are treated differently, and that in many cases this was strongly influenced by cultural issues. For example, black African and black Caribbean patients are more likely to be detained under the 1983 Mental Health Act than white patients (Davies et al., 1996) and patients from an ethnic minority community (African-Caribbean and Asian) are more likely to be admitted to secure forensic psychiatric services (Coid et al., 2000). Therefore, ethnic and cultural differences need to be incorporated within the risk assessments of people from different backgrounds.

There is also a particular concern regarding language, because for a minority of in-patients English will not be their first language, and the provision and access to interpreters in many units and trusts is variable (SCMH, 2000). This problem is significant in terms of involving patients in decisions about their care, and informing them of what their care may involve and the reasons for any decisions made. It is also essential that people from ethnic minority communities receive care that is sensitive to their cultural and religious backgrounds. Particularly with regard to observation, the gender or cultural background of a nurse observing a patient from a different cultural or religious background, may make the patient feel uneasy because of their particular beliefs or values. Such issues can be addressed through training and other activities aimed to raise staff's awareness and understanding of the religious and cultural needs of ethnic minority patients (SCMH, 2000).

Are there alternatives to observation?

Some commentators have called for a review of the practice of observation *per se* because they believe that observing patients has become primarily a custodial task rather than a therapeutic intervention (Barker and Cutcliffe, 1999; Dodds and Bowles, 2001). Indeed Barker and Cutcliffe (1999: 11) commented

> despite the rhetoric of 'supportive observation', the nurse is often construed as a custodian, if not simply the doorman.

It is indisputable that a mechanistic approach to the observation of patients at risk, which may be seen as 'watching doors' or 'guarding the patient' is totally inadequate (CRAG/SCOTMEG, 1995). However, in many places this is the reality of the practice of observation.

At the present time there are no proven effective alternatives to observation, as no large-scale randomised control study has been conducted to compare the effectiveness of observation with another suicide prevention intervention. However, there are different kinds of evidence that can be considered. Nick Bowles, Peter Dodds and their colleagues have been working in an inner-city male in-patient admission ward in Bradford, England, since 1998, to try and change observation and nursing practice on the ward. They felt that the practice of observation was

... a hidden contributory factor to the rotten state of acute admission wards that can be changed by clinicians. (Bowles and Dodds, 2001: 18)

In response they conducted a structured programme of change to observation and nursing practice as a whole, in a 'refocusing' practice development project in which they reported how the project significantly reduced the use of observation. This occurred alongside a process of more structured and individualised activity for patients, involving greater patient/staff contact and engagement, leading them to be better informed and more involved in their care. A key principle that underpinned this work was 'the gift of time' which was valued highly by the patients (Jackson and Stevenson, 1998). In addition, following the implementation of this project there have been significant reductions in: incidents of deliberate self-harm; incidents of violence and aggression; absconding; and staff sickness. There have also been financial savings by employing fewer agency and bank staff.

The work of Bowles, Dodds and their colleagues is considered by many to be innovative and to demonstrate good practice. It is important to remember that one must be cautious of making generalisations from such a small case-study; however, the achievements in Bradford demonstrate that the practice of observation cannot be changed in isolation. In order to reduce the use of observation, the nursing team, with support of the rest of the multidisciplinary team, totally reorganised the 'culture' of patient care and nursing practice on the ward. This highlights the fact that if practice is to be challenged and improved, it has to involve a cultural shift within the clinical team. This type of change is the greatest challenge of all, but it is clearly needed to turn around the poor state of acute in-patient care in the UK.

Nurses' and patients' experiences of observation

The fact that there is a dearth of research on observation *per se* has already been highlighted. There are even fewer studies that consider the nurses' and patients' perspectives of observation. This section will provide an overview of these studies, and highlight the main findings relevant to practice.

Nurses' experiences

Most studies that consider nurses' experiences about observation are small-scale and qualitative, offering a depth of understanding of some of the difficulties faced by nurses when conducting observation. Duffy (1995) conducted semi-structured interviews with 10 nurses in one in-patient unit in England. All of the nurses had experience of observing suicidal patients and the interviews disclosed a number of problematic issues for nurses who conducted the special observation procedure (the term used by Duffy). These focused on the professional autonomy of nurses, patient autonomy and paternalism. Regarding the professional autonomy of nurses, the interviews revealed that where the decision-making regarding the observation of patients remained with medical staff, then nurses would often covertly modify the doctor's orders, in a similar way to that described by Aidroos (1986). With regard to patient autonomy, the study showed an inherent tension between the paternalistic activity of preventing self-harm and the nurses' humanistic aspirations to help patients and find ways to restore their autonomy as individuals. This study also highlighted that official observation policies frequently failed to reflect the complexity and subtlety of observation, not recognising the procedure as 'a vital function of the skilled psychiatric nurse' (Duffy, 1995: 950).

Using a questionnaire survey, Reid and Long (1993) asked 45 psychiatric nurses in a hospital in Northern Ireland about their views regarding the role of the nurse in providing therapeutic care for suicidal patients. The main finding from this survey was that the nurses felt the use of special observation (authors' terminology) was the most effective preventative method in nursing suicidal patients, but they also expressed the view that the procedure was not therapeutic. Phillips et al. (1977) also found that the majority of nurses (75%) who responded to a questionnaire survey conducted in a Canadian hospital considered the procedure of continuous observation (authors' terminology) to be unsatisfactory, in terms of it being a custodial rather than therapeutic intervention.

Many nurses describe observation as a stressful and an unrewarding activity (Younge and Stewin, 1992; Cleary et al., 1999). Nurses interviewed by Cleary et al. (1999) found it difficult to act in a way that was intrusive towards patients, and they felt that this could sometimes cause some patients to become 'angry' and 'lash out'. Nurses found it particularly difficult when they were required to observe patients attending to their personal hygiene (e.g., having showers or baths) and also when they were using the lavatory. Indeed, this is a particular time when nurses will try to withdraw if at all possible (Younge and Stewin, 1992; Duffy, 1995). However, when the risks were thought to be too great, nurses set aside patients' rights to privacy and dignity, on the grounds of safety; a difficult and stressful decision to make (Bowers and Park, 2001).

Patients' experiences

Perhaps the most significant research focusing on the patient's perspective are two studies conducted in the USA. Pitula and Cardell (1996) reported a study that explored 14 suicidal in-patients' experiences of being constantly observed. This qualitative study found that the interpersonal aspect of constant observation was important, with supportive interactions with staff enhancing respondents' feelings of safety and hope. However, respondents also reported that when there was a lack of support from observers, this adversely affected their experience of observation, as did the frequent changing of observers. This has been expanded upon in a subsequent study by Cardell and Pitula (1999). Here a further 20 suicidal in-patients were interviewed to explore the possible therapeutic benefits of constant observation. It was found that therapeutic benefits from observation, such as gaining emotional support, optimism and feeling protected, were enhanced when observers had a positive attitude and engaged the participants in supportive interaction. Non-therapeutic aspects of observation were described as observers' lack of empathy, lack of acknowledgement and failure to provide information about constant observation, as well as a lack of privacy and a feeling of confinement. The clear message from these two studies is that the attitudes and behaviour of the observers seems to determine either positive or negative experiences for the patients being observed.

In the UK, Moorhead et al. (1996) surveyed 68 patients in two hospitals in the Midlands by means of a brief questionnaire. They found that 56% of respondents perceived changes in the intensity of their observation and 45% said that being observed caused discomfort. However, the scope of this study was limited and patients were not asked specifically about how being observed intensely by nurses actually made them feel. Finally, in a pilot study conducted by Jones and her colleagues, the experiences of psychiatric in-patients who were observed closely by nurses in one mental health care trust in England were explored. This study used two methods to interview patients: semi-structured interviews with 10 in-patients (Jones et al., 2000a) and the repertory grid technique with a further 18 in-patients (Jones et al., 2000b). The main finding of this research is the importance of the therapeutic relationship between nurses and patients during the intervention of nursing observation. In a positive sense, the patients interviewed said they gained a sense of security and support from the presence of nurses who were prepared to engage with them. However, more negative than positive experiences were expressed by respondents, relating in particular to the lack of information provided and the lack of supportive interaction between nurses and the patients interviewed. These findings are thus consistent with the results of other studies (Pitula and Cardell, 1996; Cardell and Pitula, 1999; Conway, 1999).

Studies comparing nurses' and patients' views

There have been a few small-scale studies conducted in the UK which have considered both the perceptions of nursing staff and patients.

Fletcher (1999) employed an ethnographic approach to compare the perceptions of 12 nursing staff who conducted constant observation with those of 6 patients who were placed on constant observation for suicidal risk. The study found a degree of commonality between the two groups; for example, with regard to the purpose of constant observation to prevent harm to patients. However, there were also interesting anomalies between the nurses and patients; for example, sitting outside a patient's room was considered by nurses to be therapeutic whereas patients considered it to be a controlling action. The majority of both positive and negative feelings on the part of patients were attributed to staff actions. Similarly, Ashaye et al. (1997) interviewed 13 patients and their respective primary nurses, in two different hospitals in the south of England, about their experiences of constant observation. The main findings were that most of the patients considered they had benefited from being on constant observation, although they disliked the intrusion on their privacy.

Observation can be stressful for both nurses and patients. By asking the people who are actually being observed as well as those doing the observing, these studies have provided a valuable insight into this activity. Generally, nurses' and patients' views on the therapeutic use of observation are similar. Patients want to be observed by nurses who treat them as people with problems, rather than simply as a diagnosis, and nurses want to engage in a therapeutic relationship, rather than act as a custodian.

Conclusion

The issues identified in this chapter highlight some of the very real problems, dilemmas and challenges faced by nurses who care for patients at risk on acute in-patient wards. It is highly problematic that there is no real 'evidence base' for the effective practice of observation, and that the written guidance that does exist has not been effectively evaluated. There are two main reasons for this. First, there is a paucity of research on observation to provide reliable research 'evidence' on how to effectively conduct observation. Second, the written guidance that has been produced, specifically the SNMAC practice guidance (DoH, 1999b) and the CRAG/SCOTMEG (1995) good-practice statement, has yet to be evaluated. Thus however sensible (or not) this guidance may seem, there is no real evidence that this guidance will improve the care of people who are observed by nurses when they are acutely ill at risk of harm.

It has been identified that even when there are local policies for observation in place, the actual practice of observation by nurses may deviate from any 'official' policy. This may be due to staff being trained inadequately and unsupported when conducting observation. However, when nurses conduct observation, they are caring for an individual person who has individual needs. Thus many nurses prefer to use their clinical judgement and experience, particularly when the needs of a person being observed may change from hour to hour, something that a prescribed doctor's order made a day before may not usefully accommodate. Indeed this is the real crux of the problem that psychiatric nursing continues to wrestle with regarding observation. There is a perceived need for guidance in the form of an evidence-based policy for observation to apply to the care of all patients at risk. However, having such fixed and objective criteria does not sit easily with a central focus on the nurse–patient relationship (Peplau, 1952) and meeting the ever-changing needs of the individual patient.

Finally, to return to the death of Sarah Kane. It is clear from the findings of the *Report of the National Confidential Inquiry into Suicide and Homicide by People with Mental Illness* (DoH, 2001) that better suicide prevention is needed for the population as a whole, and that suicides by in-patients are seen as the most preventable. We also know from the findings of the report that in-patients continue to commit suicide when they are officially being observed. It seems imperative that the whole practice of observation must be reviewed, in conjunction with acute in-patient care as a whole. This is all too late for Sarah Kane, whose life was lost due to her illness and the lack of care provided by the mental health system, but we must retain hope that things will improve, and that more people will be kept safe in a way that is both supportive and therapeutic.

Acknowledgements

We wish to thank Nigel Wellman and Trevor Lowe for their helpful comments on an earlier draft of this chapter.

References

Aidroos, N. (1986) 'Nurses' response to doctors' orders for close observation', *Canadian Journal of Psychiatry*, 31: 831–3.

Allen, J. (1998) 'Acute admission psychiatric nursing', *Journal of Psychiatric and Mental Health Nursing*, 5 (5): 427–9.

Appleby, L., Shaw, J., Amos, T., McDonnell, R., Harris, C., McCann, K., Kiernan, K., Davies, S., Bickley, H. and Parsons, R. (1999) 'Suicide within 12 months of contact with mental health services: national clinical survey', *British Medical Journal*, 318: 1235–9.

Ashaye, O., Ikkos, G. and Rigby, E. (1997) 'Study of effects of constant observation of psychiatric in-patients', *Psychiatric Bulletin* 21: 145–7.

Barker, P. and Cutcliffe, J. (1999) 'Clinical risk: a need for engagement not observation', *Mental Health Practice*, 2 (8): 8–12.

Bowers, L. and Park, A. (2001) 'Special observation in the care of psychiatric inpatients: a literature review', *Issues in Mental Health Nursing*, 22: 769–86.

Bowers, L., Gournay, K. and Duffy, D. (2000) 'Suicide and self-harm in inpatient psychiatric units: a national survey of observation policies', *Journal of Advanced Nursing*, 32 (2): 437–44.

Bowles, N. and Dodds, P. (2001) 'Eye for an eye', *Openmind*, 108: 18–19.

Cardell, R. and Pitula, C.R. (1999) 'Suicidal inpatients' perceptions of therapeutic and nontherapeutic aspects of constant observation', *Psychiatric Services*, 50: 1066–70.

Childs, A., Thomas, B. and Tibbles, P. (1994) 'Specialist needs', *Nursing Times*, 90 (3): 32–3.

Cleary, M., Jordan, R., Horsfall, J., Mazoudier, P. and Delaney, J. (1999) 'Suicidal patients and special observation', *Journal of Psychiatric and Mental Health Nursing*, 6: 461–7.

Coid, J., Kahtan, N., Gault, S. and Jarman, B. (2000) 'Ethnic differences in admissions to secure psychiatric services', *British Journal of Psychiatry*, 177: 241–7.

Conway, E.A. (1999) 'A multi-dimensional study of the process of observation in acute mental health wards, involving policy documentation, staff and user views', Report to Newcastle City Health Trust, Newcastle.

CRAG/SCOTMEG (Working Group on Mental Illness) (1995) *Nursing Observation of Acutely Ill Psychiatric Patients in Hospital: A Good Practice Statement*. Edinburgh: The Scottish Office.

Davies, S., Thornicroft, G., Leese, M., Higgingbotham, A. and Phelan, M. (1996) 'Ethnic differences in risk of compulsory psychiatric admission among representative cases of psychosis in London', *British Medical Journal*, 312 (7030): 533–7.

Dennis, S. (1997) 'Close observation: how to improve assessments', *Nursing Times*, 93 (24): 54–6.

Department of Health (1999a) *Report by the Standing Nursing and Midwifery Advisory Committee (SNMAC). Mental Health Nursing: Addressing Acute Concerns*. London: The Stationery Office.

Department of Health (1999b) *Practice Guidance: Safe and Supportive Observation of Patients at Risk. Mental Health Nursing: Addressing Acute Concerns*. London: The Stationery Office.

Department of Health (1999c) *A National Service Framework for Mental Health*. London: The Stationery Office.

Department of Health (2001) *Safety First: Five-Year Report of the National Confidential Inquiry into Suicide and Homicide by People with Mental Illness*. London: The Stationery Office.

Dodds, P. and Bowles, N. (2001) 'Dismantling formal observation and refocusing nursing activity in acute inpatient psychiatry: a case study', *Journal of Psychiatric and Mental Health Nursing*, 8: 183–8.

Duffy, D. (1995) 'Out of the shadows: a study of the special observation of suicidal psychiatric in-patients', *Journal of Advanced Nursing*, 21 (5): 944–50.

Fletcher, R.F. (1999) 'The process of constant observation: perspectives of staff and suicidal patients', *Journal of Psychiatric Mental Health Nursing*, 6 (1): 9–14.

Guardian (1999) 'Suicidal writer was free to kill herself', *The Guardian*, 23 September, pp. 4–5.

Higgins, R., Hurst, K. and Wistow, G. (1999) *Psychiatric Care Revisited: The Care Provided for Acute Psychiatric Patients*. London: Whurr.

Jackson, S. and Stevenson, C. (1998) 'The gift of time from the friendly professional', *Nursing Standard*, 12 (51): 31–3.

Jones, J., Lowe, T. and Ward, M. (2000a) 'Inpatients' experiences of nursing observation on an acute psychiatric unit: a pilot study', *Mental Health Care*, 4 (4): 125–9.

Jones, J., Ward, M., Wellman, N., Hall, J. and Lowe, T. (2000b) 'Psychiatric inpatients' experiences of nursing observation – a UK perspective', *Journal of Psychosocial Nursing and Mental Health Services*, 38 (12): 10–20.

Kettles, A. (2000) Personal communication with the authors.

Kettles, A. (2001) 'The relationship between self-harming behaviour and the level of observation patients are placed on at the time of admission: an exploratory study', Presentation at the 7th International NPNR Conference, Oxford, September.

Midence, K., Gregory, S. and Rea, S. (1996) 'The effects of patient suicide on staff', *Journal of Clinical Nursing*, 5: 115–20.

Moore, P., Berman, K., Knight, M. and Devine, J. (1995) 'Constant observation: implications for nursing practice', *Journal of Psychosocial Nursing*, 33 (3): 46–50.

Moorhead, S.M.L., Kennedy, J., Hodgson, C.M., Ruiz, P. and Junaid, O. (1996) 'Observations of the observed: a study of inpatients' perception of being observed', *Irish Journal of Psychological Medicine*, 13 (2): 59–61.

Neilson, P. and Brennan, W. (2001) 'The use of special observations: an audit within a psychiatric unit', *Journal of Psychiatric and Mental Health Nursing*, 8: 147–55.

Peplau, H.E. (1952) *Interpersonal Relations in Nursing*. London: Macmillan.

Phillips, M., Peacocke, J., Hermanstyne, L., Rosales, A., Rowe, M., Smith, P., Steele, C. and Weaver, R. (1977) 'Continuous observation – Part 1', *Canadian Psychiatric Association*, 22: 25–8.

Pitula, C.R. and Cardell, R. (1996) 'Suicidal inpatients' experience of constant observation', *Psychiatric Services*, 47 (6): 649–51.

Porter, S., McCann, I. and Kettles, M.A. (1998) 'Auditing suicide observation procedures', *Psychiatric Care*, 1: 17–21.

Reid, W. and Long, A. (1993) 'The role of the nurse providing therapeutic care for the suicidal patient', *Journal of Advanced Nursing*, 18: 1369–76.

Ritter, S. (1989) *Bethlem Royal and Maudsley Hospitals Manual of Clinical Psychiatric Nursing Principles and Procedures*. London: Harper & Row.

Sainsbury Centre for Mental Health (SCMH) (1997) *The National Visit*. London: Mental Health Act Commission/Sainsbury Centre for Mental Health.

Sainsbury Centre for Mental Health (SCMH) (1998) *Acute Problems: A Survey of the Quality of Care in Acute Psychiatric Wards*. London: Sainsbury Centre for Mental Health.

Sainsbury Centre for Mental Health (SCMH) (2000) *The National Visit 2: Improving Care for Detained Patients from Black and Minority Ethnic Communities*. London: Sainsbury Centre for Mental Health.

Shugar, G. and Rehaluk, R. (1990) 'Continuous observation for psychiatric inpatients: a critical evaluation', *Comprehensive Psychiatry*, 31 (1): 48–55.

Ward, M., Gournay, K., Thornicroft, G. and Wright, S. (1998) *In-Patient Mental Health Services in Inner London: 1997 Census*. Oxford: Royal College of Nursing Institute.

Younge, O. and Stewin, L.L. (1992) 'What psychiatric nurses say about constant care', *Clinical Nursing Research*, 1 (1): 80–90.

NINE

Cognitive behaviour therapy in in-patient care

Kevin Gournay

Introduction

As the reader may know, the author of this chapter led the research team, which provided the underpinning work for the report *Addressing Acute Concerns* (SNMAC, 1999). Following a sounding board event, the research team carried out a literature review and policy analysis and followed that up with specific work on management of violence and observation. During the course of the work, it became clear that there was a dearth of evidence-based therapeutic interventions provided to patients in in-patient environments. Overall, our work painted a picture of services which provided a reasonable degree of safety and asylum, but very little by way of therapeutic interventions. The picture obtained by the research team in the late 1990s really was no different to that which faced the Clinical Standards Advisory Group (CSAG), who examined a representative sample of services in an attempt to provide a picture of care provided to people with schizophrenia in the UK several years before. Eventually, CSAG published its report (DoH, 1995) and made clear recommendations about the need to provide therapeutic rather than custodial interventions. Sadly, there seems to have been little progress between the Clinical Standards Advisory Group work and *Addressing Acute Concerns*.

This chapter focuses on the application of evidence-based therapeutic interventions, particularly cognitive behaviour therapy within the in-patient setting. The primary purpose of this chapter is to provide the clinical nurse with an account of this approach and to provide an overview of cognitive behavioural procedures, which would be useful to clinical nurses in everyday NHS settings. This chapter, while it will refer to research and cognitive behaviour theory, is not meant to be a theoretical discussion, or indeed, a scientific critique. Hopefully, at the end of the chapter, the reader will be able to appreciate some of the underpinning theory and overall should be equipped with some of the basic knowledge which is necessary to develop cognitive behavioural skills. The chapter will include the following sections.

- The basis of cognitive behaviour therapy (CBT) and its application within the in-patient setting.
- CBT: a longstanding tradition in nursing.
- The CBT framework (including measurement and experimentation).
- Specific cognitive behavioural techniques.
- Summary.
- Conclusion.

The basis of cognitive behaviour therapy (CBT) and its application within the in-patient setting

While the term cognitive behaviour therapy (CBT) is very well known now to most mental health professionals, it might be worth (by way of introduction) describing how this current concept has evolved. The roots and origins of CBT go back to the turn of the 20th century when various behavioural psychologists began to develop various theories of learning. As most readers will know, Ivan Pavlov, a Russian psychologist, was foremost in this movement, and most nursing students will have read about Pavlov's work with dogs and conditioned reflexes. Similarly, the behavioural theories of Skinner, which were developed in the 1930s and 1940s, focused on learning by reinforcement, and this work was originally applied in educational settings. Once more, most nursing students will have received a basic introduction to operant conditioning and other 'Skinnerian' concepts. I will not therefore reiterate the history of learning theories, other than to say that it is important to recognise that the theories relating to classical conditioning and operant conditioning originally underpinned some of the later treatment approaches which became known as behaviour therapy.

Behaviour therapy for neurotic problems developed from the learning theory approaches in the 1950s. A South African psychiatrist (who had settled in the USA), Joseph Wolpe, developed treatments based on classical conditioning theories. Wolpe's work led to the first treatments of phobias by a process known as *systematic desensitisation*. In this approach Wolpe coupled with the anxiety stimulus, another stimulus which was incompatible with anxiety, a process known as reciprocal inhibition. In practice, Wolpe taught patients to relax in association with presenting them with images of the things they feared. Thus, in graduated doses of difficulty, Wolpe successfully treated many patients with phobias. During the late 1960s and early 1970s, systematic desensitisation was replaced by a more practical form of treatment known as graduated exposure, something to which we will refer below, as it has become very important to specialist mental health nursing. Other forms of behaviour therapy, based on classical conditioning, were developed primarily for the treatment of people with conditions known as neuroses, or today more commonly called 'common mental disorders'. Thus behaviour therapy was widened to include treatments for obsessive compulsive disorder, social phobias and sexual problems. For a more detailed account of these developments in nursing, see Newell and Gournay (2000).

With regard to treatments for serious and enduring mental illnesses such as schizophrenia, the learning theories of Skinner provided the basis for other developments. The first clinical applications of this approach were made in the 1950s and 1960s,when American psychologists used Skinner's theories as a basis for treating patients with chronic schizophrenia. These developments, largely based in the USA, led to the now legendary token economy units (Ayllon and Azrin, 1968). Token economies were essentially in-patient units where staff/patient ratios were very high, often one to one. Following very detailed assessment, patients were subjected to treatment, which focused on a number of 'socially desirable behaviours'. Thus, the common problems which one sees in chronic schizophrenia, such as lack of motivation, poor daily living skills and social withdrawal, were targeted. The programme worked 24 hours a day and all socially desirable behaviours were reinforced by giving the patient tokens. These tokens normally took the form of discs, which were carried in pouches by the nursing staff. Each time the patient performed a behaviour, which was on the target list, the patient was immediately reinforced by the nurse who gave the token. At the end of the day, the patient could exchange the tokens for a wide range of rewards, including tobacco, sweets and additional food, or the patient could save the tokens to buy extra privileges such as leave outside the wards. In the UK, token economy systems were developed in specialist units during the 1970s, the most well known of which were in Wakefield, Yorkshire, and Hellingly, Sussex. In these hospitals, the staffing ratios were very high and while the patient was on the unit, progress was often very dramatic. However, when they were discharged to the community or to other more ordinary wards in the hospital, the treatment gains were often quickly lost. Nevertheless, it became clear that the approach could be used as an intensive 'quick start' for a rehabilitation process. Unfortunately, because of the expense of running such highly staffed units, and the additional expenses for staff training and rehabilitation resources, the use of the token economy drifted into oblivion. Nevertheless, this development (although this is not widely recognised now) was very influential in contemporary applications of behaviour and cognitive behavioural techniques. Thus, from the systematic desensitisation and token economy systems, behaviour therapy evolved and various treatments were developed which included strands from both classical and operant conditioning. By the late 1970s, the links between pragmatically developed treatment approaches and the detailed psychological theories became weakened however. One of the central reasons for this was the increasing recognition that nurses (who did not have any detailed grounding in psychological theory) could apply behavioural treatments equally well, as highly trained (and expensive) clinical psychologists. In addition, it also became clear that the treatments themselves were becoming divorced from the previously used rigid applications of behavioural theory, and effective treatment approaches could not be explained in terms of pure psychological theory. Given what we now know, about the basis of mental illness – i.e., that most mental illnesses have biological, psychological and social origins – this is not surprising.

In recent times, the most important development has been the integration of cognitive approaches with behavioural approaches to form what is now known as cognitive behaviour therapy (CBT). This work is attributed to the American psychiatrist Aaron Beck, who tested approaches which were loosely based on trying to teach the patient to think more rationally and to change faulty patterns of thinking. CBT techniques have been applied to a range of mental health problems, but principally to address the negative patterns of thinking that are associated with depression. Indeed, virtually all of the large-scale research conducted on cognitive therapy during the 1980s and early 1990s was on patients with depression and predominantly on those treated as out-patients.

It is worth noting, however, that one of the early applications of CBT was with a patient suffering from chronic schizophrenia (Beck, 1952). This has been reflected over the last decade where CBT has become associated with a wide range of other mental health problems, from fears and phobias to the most severe forms of mental illness including schizophrenia and severe personality disorder.

CBT: a longstanding tradition in nursing

As previously noted, during the late 1960s and early 1970s behaviour therapy was developed from the systematic desensitisation approaches invented by Joseph Wolpe. These early developments led to techniques such as exposure therapy for phobias and response prevention for obsessive compulsive disorder to evolve as effective treatments (Newell and Gournay, 2000). However, it became clear that whilst these treatments provided a great deal of hope for ameliorating previously intractable distress suffered by literally hundreds of thousands of individuals, the workforce available to treat these conditions amounted to no more than a few dozen psychologists and psychiatrists. In this setting, the psychiatrist Isaac Marks, who worked at the Institute of Psychiatry and Maudsley Hospital, identified nurses as being the most suitable workforce to deliver these interventions. In 1972, Marks commenced a three-year pilot programme, which trained five nurses to become behaviour therapists, principally in the treatment of anxiety and related disorders. This was the first programme to train nurses to become independent therapists, although since that time there have been several hundred nurses trained. Nurse therapists now deliver cognitive behaviour therapy for a range of common mental disorders, including obsessive compulsive states, post-traumatic stress disorder, simple phobias, social phobia and agoraphobia.

Since the setting up of the original nurse therapy programme, there have been several attempts to develop these skills in nurses working in in-patient settings. However, these efforts have largely been unsuccessful. The report *Addressing Acute Concerns* (SNMAC, 1999) recognised that patients receiving in-patient care are, by and large, not being availed of evidence-based psychological treatment approaches. Given the great shortage of clinical psychologists (only about 3,000 in the UK), it seems clear that nurses represent a very suitable workforce for delivering evidence-based psychological interventions. Given the example of the nurse therapy programme for treating common mental disorders, there seems no reason why similar training programmes should not be set up which focus on psychological treatments for conditions such as schizophrenia and applied in both in-patient and community settings.

The CBT framework

Possibly because of the associations of the early behavioural approaches with the conditioning of animals, there was in the past (and still is to some extent), the belief that behavioural and cognitive behavioural approaches somehow lack a humane dimension. While it is true that the approaches do rely on the application of a scientific approach and that some of the treatment approaches are based on theories of learning derived from animal experiments, cognitive behaviour therapy is based on building a collaborative relationship with the patient. There is a great deal of emphasis on seeing the patient's problems in a very individualistic way, and the cognitive behavioural assessment process includes a great emphasis on understanding how the problem has developed in that particular individual. It is therefore important for the therapist to understand how the person sees themselves, their problem and the world about them. Another very important part of the assessment process involves identifying the patient's strengths and coping mechanisms, so that these may be used to good advantage during the treatment process. Overall, therefore, the approach (if applied correctly) is undoubtedly collaborative, and the therapist's role is to help patients help themselves. Therefore, at each stage of the assessment process, the therapist validates their understanding of the problem within the patient and suggests a range of techniques and strategies which the patient can use.

Measurement

In general health care, it is very important to measure the extent of the patient's physical problem. With a problem such as hypertension, one obviously needs to measure blood pressure. Similarly with diabetes, blood sugar is a central measure. However, with these conditions, there are other components of the person's physical health and well-being which also require measurement. Consequently, for someone with high blood pressure, one might also want to measure kidney function, cardiac function or, in an advanced case, cognitive function to check whether the brain has been affected by the longstanding effects on the fragile blood vessels of the brain.

Traditionally, mental health workers have been very poor at measuring patients' mental health or illnesses. Even now, most patients with depression do not have their mood measured with valid and reliable tools such as the Beck Depression Inventory (Beck, 1952). If the problem being targeted is not measured, it is very difficult to establish whether treatment is having an effect.

In many ways mental health problems are more complex than physical problems such as high blood pressure or diabetes. For example, while someone with schizophrenia may have problems which are characterised by positive and negative symptoms, there are also a wide range of other problems such as the effects on the family, the patient's quality of life and their ability to take part in normal daily living processes. Thus mental health problems should be measured as broadly as possible, using not only indices of the central problem (for example, the positive and negative symptoms) but also including aspects such as family burden, met and unmet needs and social functioning. It is inappropriate to provide a list of tools or measures in this chapter; however, it is worth noting that there are relatively brief, but effective, measures which can be used after relatively short training programmes. For example, in the Thorn programme, which is primarily aimed at staff working in community settings, students are trained to use measures of met and unmet needs such as the Camberwell

Assessment of Need (Phelan et al., 1995) or the standardised psychiatric assessment for chronic psychotic patients (Krawiecka et al., 1977).

Measurements should be taken using established, valid and reliable tools that examine various facets of the patient's problem and identify improvement in some or all aspects. One may generally expect a patient with depression to recover to the extent that all measurable areas improve. However, with a patient with chronic schizophrenia, one may observe improvement only in some areas. Consequently, cognitive behavioural measures should include general measures such as social functioning. However, they must also include very specific measures of change.

Experimentation

Experimentation is a core characteristic of the cognitive behavioural approach. There is often a range of techniques which may be of benefit to patients with specific problems. For example, in depression, one might use cognitive techniques to help the patient change a particularly negative thought. However, in addition, the therapist will know that for some patients, specific exercises are important. Some patients may benefit from using a timetabling approach to structuring their activities while others benefit from training in improving assertive skills and others from the use of medication and so on. The cognitive behavioural approach requires the therapist to develop a programme of treatment, which incorporates the use of a number of techniques. However, as each patient responds in their own individual way, one needs to find the optimum technique or combination of techniques. This can only be done by actually trying the techniques (singularly or in combination) in real life. Thus, in a sense, each trial of treatment becomes an experiment in its own right. The therapist should use a range of measures before applying the techniques, and again after the application, in order to ascertain the effectiveness of these techniques. Then, once the therapist has had the opportunity to consider the results of the measures and to discuss the outcome with the patient, the techniques and strategies can be varied. This approach, combining measurement and experimentation with clinical practice, is often called the approach of the 'scientist practitioner'.

Finally, the cognitive behavioural approach relies on the application of evidence (obtained from research) to practice. The cognitive behavioural framework assumes that the person who delivers the cognitive behaviour approach has a broad knowledge of the scientific literature relating to research on the efficacy of various procedures and techniques. Thus, for example, the knowledgeable practitioner of cognitive behaviour therapy should know which approaches work and which approaches do not work for various problems. Although this seems rather obvious, it is worth noting that patients with mental health problems still receive many treatments for which there is no evidence base. Thus, it is common to see patients with phobic anxiety disorders who have been provided with psycho-analytically based treatments, (which have long since been shown to be ineffective) or patients with obsessive compulsive disorder who have been treated with counselling, or patients with psychoses who have been treated with an inappropriate combination of medications. Critically reading the papers that provide evidence is therefore very important. It is worth noting here that there are various established levels of evidence and that, if available, the practitioner should use treatment approaches proven by the highest possible level of evidence. These are as follows.

- **Level 1.** Evidence established from a number of well-designed randomised controlled trials.
- **Level 2.** Evidence from at least one properly designed randomised controlled trial.
- **Level 3.** Evidence from well-designed controlled trials without randomisation.
- **Level 4.** Well-designed case-controlled or other quasi-experimental studies.
- **Level 5.** Non-experimental descriptive studies.
- **Level 6.** Expert reports and opinions of respected authorities.

It needs to be said that in in-patient care the evidence is very poor because of the lack of investment of research with in-patient populations. Thus, there is very little evidence at levels 1, 2 and 3, which contrasts greatly with areas such as anxiety disorders where there are literally thousands of randomised controlled trials to testify to the effectiveness of various treatment approaches.

Specific cognitive behavioural techniques

In order to provide an overview of these techniques, it is easiest to consider the problem areas where these techniques are applied. While one needs to assume that most in-patients have problems which come under the umbrella of severe and enduring mental illnesses, it is also worth noting that many people with severe mental illnesses, such as schizophrenia, also have problems with anxiety and depression: the so-called 'minor' mental disorders. The following descriptions of approach therefore include an emphasis on areas in treating such problems.

1. Increasing activity.
2. Learning new behaviour.

3. Changing cognitive processes.
4. Dealing with anxiety.
5. Dealing with depression.

Increasing activity

Many in-patients, particularly those with schizophrenia or severe depression, often have very reduced levels of activity. It is therefore important that staff in in-patient settings are aware of the importance of increasing the activity of patients who are particularly withdrawn, as apathy and withdrawal compound depression and helplessness. The care plan therefore needs to reflect this emphasis. Indeed, for some patients it may be important to work out an hour-to-hour timetable rather than relying on those activities that take place during the traditional 10–4 occupational therapy programme. Obviously, if ward staff are to take an active part in increasing activity, there is a need for sufficient numbers of staff to be present. However, there is no reason why family members or volunteers should not be used to ensure that patients are as fully occupied and active as possible.

Learning new behaviour

Nurses in in-patient settings are ideally placed to assist patients with the learning of new behaviour. Some examples of problems which may come under this heading are as follows:

- poor eye contact;
- deficits in verbal communication;
- deficits in non-verbal communication;
- problems with assertion;
- poor daily living skills.

The central approach to deal with these problems of social behaviour is social skills training. Although this method of treatment has not received a great deal of attention in contemporary literature, there is no doubt that it can be very effective; for example, Smith et al. (1996) reviewed nine studies of social skills training, and argued that the approach was effective for a range of problems. Smith et al. also suggested that social skills approaches, used in combination with medication, could be a very effective treatment for people with chronic schizophrenia. The approach may, however, take a great deal of time, and obviously what can be achieved in the acute ward setting is limited. Nevertheless, ward staff may be in an excellent position to make an assessment of social skills problems so that they may be targeted in the longer term, and, where appropriate, continued by community staff on discharge. There are four central components to social skills training:

- instruction;
- modelling;
- feedback;
- homework.

Instruction involves instructing the patient in a particular behaviour; to take one simple example, a patient who has poor eye contact may be instructed to attempt to try to make more eye contact, and the nurse will be able to discuss the reasons why this may be particularly beneficial.

Modelling involves helping the patient learn by observing the behaviour in someone else. Thus, if the patient is facing an interview with the Benefits Agency the nurse could demonstrate, through a process of modelling, how they should approach the situation.

Feedback, providing the patient with information about their performance. It is most important that feedback should be delivered by emphasising, first of all, what has been done well, and then providing very specific information on what needs to be improved. Simply presenting critical feedback will be very destructive. Therefore, providing the patient with reinforcement for achievement is essential.

Homework involves setting the patient tasks to do which may involve trying out a new behaviour. This is then followed by more instruction, modelling and feedback, and so on.

Changing cognitive processes

In recent years there has been considerable emphasis on using cognitive behavioural strategies to modify the delusional thinking associated with schizophrenia and other psychotic illnesses. For an excellent review of this area see Kingdon (1998). Essentially the approach should only be used by those who have received specific training in CBT. However, new training programmes for in-patient nurses are now including these strategies. Cognitive behavioural approaches to modify delusions involves a detailed assessment process, followed by a very systematic challenging of the delusional beliefs. The approach is collaborative, not confrontational, and the therapist works with the patient to look at the delusion in various ways. It does seem that, with some patients, this approach weakens delusional thinking considerably. A similar approach is used with auditory hallucinations, which are so common in schizophrenia, and often cause the patient considerable distress. Working with the patient in a detailed and systematic way can lead to better coping and the cognitive behavioural approach involves helping the patient understand how the hallucinations have developed, and to put them within the context of the illness. Sometimes helping patients to understand particular triggers for hallucinations enables them to approach triggering situations differently, thus modifying the onset of the hallucinations. Simple techniques such as distraction, or masking the hallucination by use of a personal hi-fi may also be effective. As with delusions the approach is collaborative; however, while these approaches are not very complex, they often take a great deal of time to implement.

Dealing with anxiety

Although the majority of patients in acute wards have psychotic illnesses, many also have symptoms of anxiety. Because the symptoms of the primary disorder often dominate the clinical picture, though, often the symptoms of anxiety are either not detected or, if they are detected, they are seen as very much secondary to the central problem. It should therefore be remembered that people with severe mental illnesses are just as entitled to suffer anxiety as anyone else! In the ward setting the staff may be able to play a very valuable part in reducing patients' anxiety and this may be achieved at three levels:

- physiological;
- cognitive;
- behavioural.

Physiologically anxiety may be reduced by simple relaxation training and, in the busy ward environment, if nursing staff do not have sufficient time, there are many good commercially available tapes which may be used by the patient under minimal supervision. Physical exercise is another simple strategy, which will reduce physiological arousal, and is perhaps of more general benefit, particularly in the restrictive environments of in-patient care where patients' access to exercise is not readily available.

Cognitive approaches help the patient by talking through their central fears and consider the rationality of their beliefs and consequences. For a more detailed account of simple anxiety reduction strategies see Gournay (1996).

Behaviourally patients may be helped to reduce avoidance behaviour and face their feared situations. The simple principle here is that one should make a careful assessment of the patient's avoidance behaviours and, in collaboration with the patient, construct a list of situations, which the patient should then confront. Tackling this list in 'graduated doses of difficulty' is very important, and the patient should feel that they are facing their fears in a way that is manageable for them. Once more there are limitations to what can be achieved in an in-patient setting, but this may represent the beginning of a programme of very positive therapeutic change.

Dealing with depression

Depressive symptoms are very common in the in-patient population, and their distress may be greatly relieved by the prescription of an appropriate medication. However, there is clear evidence that depression may be effectively treated by cognitive behavioural therapy provided either alone or in conjunction with the appropriate drug (Stuart, 2001). The cognitive behavioural approach involves a number of steps. First of all there is a need to carry out a very detailed assessment of particular thoughts, triggers for these thoughts and detailed content of those thoughts. The therapist may then be able to help the patient challenge assumptions about themselves and the world in general, and using a systematic process begin to teach the patient new ways of thinking. CBT is usually provided by a specialist nurse therapist or clinical psychologist. However, contemporary training programmes are emphasising the role of ward staff in assisting with this approach. Perhaps the most valuable contribution that ward staff can make is in the assessment process. Through the therapeutic relationship between ward staff and patient, information about the nature and content of the depressive thoughts may be collected as it is only by obtaining such a detailed account that the patient may be helped to change.

Summary

CBT is a broad group of approaches which are effective in reducing a number of psychiatric conditions. While it is not expected that all in-patient staff should be specialist practitioners of CBT methods, it is important that they should understand its principles and how it may be applied in in-patient settings.

Conclusion

Nurses have used cognitive behavioural techniques for nearly 30 years, and the nurse therapist was probably the first example of the autonomous nurse practitioner. Until very recently, though, nursing and cognitive behavioural approaches have been confined to community settings. It is now clear that cognitive behavioural approaches can be helpful with many in-patients. Staff in such settings should therefore have a basic understanding of how these approaches are applied, and while not expecting all nurses to have higher-level skills in this area, it seems clear that there is a role for specialist nurse practitioners working with in-patients. If such roles do not develop it is likely that the largely custodial environments, which dominate in today's acute in-patient units, will continue to exist. Making in-patient care more therapeutic is an aspiration which will rely almost entirely on the skills of nurses in providing therapeutic techniques.

References

Ayllon, T. and Azrin, N. (1968) *The Token Economy: A Motivational System for Therapy and Rehabilitation.* New York: Appleton-Century-Crofts.

Beck, A. (1952) 'Successful outpatients psychotherapy of a chronic schizophrenic with a delusion based on borrowed guilt', *Psychiatry*, 15: 305–12.

Department of Health (1995) *Clinical Standards Advisory Group: Schizophrenia*, Vol. 1. London: HMSO.

Gournay, K. (1996) *No Panic.* Dorking: Asset Books.

Kingdon, D. (1998) 'Cognitive behaviour therapy for severe mental illness; strategies and techniques', in C. Brooker and J. Repper (eds), *Serious Mental Health Problems in the Community: Policy, Practice and Research.* London: Baillière Tindall. pp. 184–203.

Krawiecka, M., Goldberg, D. and Vaughan, M. (1977) 'A standardised psychiatric assessment for chronic psychotic patients', *Acta Psychiatrica Scandinavica*, 55: 299–308.

Newell, R. and Gournay, K. (2000) *Mental Health Nursing – An Evidence Based Approach.* London: Churchill Livingstone.

Phelan, M., Slade, M. and Thornicroft, G. (1995) 'The Camberwell assessment of need', *British Journal of Psychiatry*, 167: 589–95.

Smith T., Ballack A. and Liberman, R. (1996) 'Social skills training for schizophrenia: review and future directions', *Clinical Psychology Review*, 16: 599–617.

Standing Nursing Midwifery Advisory Committee (SNMAC) (1999) *Mental Health Nursing: Addressing Acute Concerns.* London: The Stationery Office.

Stuart, G. (2001) 'Cognitive behavioural therapy', in G. Stuart, and M. Laraia (eds), *Principles and Practice of Psychiatric Nursing.* St Louis: Mosby. pp. 658–72.

TEN
Psychosocial interventions
Ian Baguley and Julie Dulson

Summary

Psychosocial interventions describe the complex activities undertaken by clinicians and services that focus upon improving the health and social situation of clients who suffer from severe mental illness (Baguley and Baguley, 1999). These interventions have been found to have positive effects for patients in terms of relapse rates (measured by admissions to hospital and outcome measurements), symptom reduction and improved social functioning (Lancashire et al., 1996).

The interventions can be split into three broad areas: early intervention and relapse planning, individual cognitive behavioural interventions for psychosis, and family interventions. This chapter describes these interventions in more detail and suggests how they can be adapted for use by nurses and other professionals working in acute in-patient areas.

Introduction

Serious and enduring mental illnesses such as schizophrenia are characterised by poor social performance, severe underemployment, higher than normal morbidity rates, high risk of suicide and self-harm and high levels of substance misuse. This gives a clear indication of the range and complexity of need that patients suffering from these illnesses are likely to have. Medication alone, despite recent developments, is often not enough to help people to meet such complex needs.

The diverse components of care required to help patients with serious mental illness requires careful coordination, the introduction of case management and the care programme approach (and later effective care co-ordination) in the UK was an attempt to manage complex care packages for clients with complex needs. Acute in-patient treatment is one component of a complex care package. This means that acute in-patient units are as much a community resource (and as important a part of a treatment package) as, say, an assertive community treatment team. Acute in-patient wards are required, therefore, to offer the highly specialised interventions to meet those complex needs.

Nursing in acute in-patient settings presents many challenges to the psychiatric nurse. Admission usually happens when the patient is acutely ill, often under a section of the Mental Health Act and frequently, along with their families and carers, distressed and upset. At the same time, services are under extreme pressure. It is not uncommon to have bed occupancy above 100%, and the constant flow of new admissions, staff shortages and diversity of patient need may further complicate this picture, often resulting in an environment that is extremely stressful to both patients and staff (MHAC/SCMH, 1997).

The Sainsbury Centre for Mental Health (1998) interviewed 112 patients at the time of their discharge from acute in-patient settings and found that these settings are eminently unpopular with patients. They found that many wards lacked basic facilities with conditions being especially poor in deprived areas. Of greater concern is the authors' findings that many patients, particularly women, felt unsafe or had concerns about their personal safety during their stay in hospital. The experience of mental illness is often a very frightening and distressing one; it is unthinkable that services add to this distress by placing people, often against their will in environments where they do not feel safe.

A lack of involvement in the planning and evaluation of their care, inadequate staff contact and a lack of something constructive to do are all concerns expressed by service users (DoH, 2002). The authors of the Sainsbury Centre's report *Acute Concerns* (SCMH, 1998) agree with these concerns, arguing that in many cases 'hospital care is a non-therapeutic intervention' (p. 41). They suggest that there are three areas or concerns that need to be addressed. First, the environment, which is often lacking in basic facilities; second, the needs of specific groups of people such as women or ethnic minorities are not being addressed; and third, the care offered is not meeting the social or therapeutic needs of clients. Whilst the lack of basic facilities is clearly a problem to be addressed by senior managers, the implementation of psychosocial interventions into acute areas will go some way in addressing the other two concerns. Psychosocial interventions are structured and collaborative; the aim is always to work from the patient's perspective and the person must be fully involved at all times. The emphasis is on engagement and normalisation (to be discussed below) and the development of a holistic approach to encompass all the person's needs.

Background

The notion that illnesses such as schizophrenia may react poorly to stress is not a new one. Lidz et al. (1957) noted that upset within the family seemed to generate stress and this was associated with a deterioration in the patient's illness.

The first link between patterns of communication and stress within the home environment was made by Bateson and his colleagues in the mid-1950s. Bateson observed that it was not always the content of what people said to the patient that was important, rather the way they said it. This led to the formulation of the double-blind hypothesis (Bateson et al., 1956) and led to the conclusion that dysfunctional patterns of communication (e.g., when a mother said something approving about a child, but indicated disapproval non-verbally), could cause an illness such as schizophrenia. Although there is no evidence to support this hypothesis, there is evidence to support the notion that patterns of communications between clients and carers may have a role to play in the amelioration of symptoms.

Research in the late 1950s and early 1960s began to examine the factors that were thought to contribute to relapse in schizophrenia, particularly the adjustment of patients following discharge from a large psychiatric hospital in London (Brown et al., 1958). Brown (1959) studied a large sub-group of these patients who had a diagnosis of schizophrenia and found that those patients who returned from hospital to live with a family or relative fared worse in terms of relapse than those patients who lived alone or in supported accommodation (Brown, 1959).

Over the next 15 years, two broad themes began to emerge from the research. First, patients who returned to live with a family where relatives exhibited a high degree of expressed emotion (HEE), which is characterised by displays of emotional over-involvement, hostility and criticism, were likely to relapse quicker than those who returned to live with relatives who displayed low expressed emotion (LEE). Second, the amount of contact time between the patient and relatives within HEE households and the patient's compliance with medication were important ameliorating factors. Those patients who spent less than 35 hours per week in direct face-to-face contact with an HEE relative and who complied with their medication relapsed less than those who had high face-to-face contact and did not comply with their medication (Leff and Vaughn, 1980; Vaughn and Leff, 1981).

Psychosocial interventions are based upon the stress vulnerability model of psychosis (Zubin and Spring, 1977). This model is suggested as a method of explaining not just the onset of psychosis but also any subsequent relapses. The model suggests that some people have a predisposition or vulnerability to develop psychosis. Once someone has experienced a first, acute, episode there is a relationship between stressors, both acute and ambient, in the person's environment that may contribute to an increase in the symptoms of psychosis.

It is suggested that the amount of stress required to produce psychotic symptoms is in inverse correlation to the amount of vulnerability that person has; i.e., the more vulnerability the less stress required to trigger an acute episode. Acute stress describes that stress that can be generated as a result of major life events such as the death of a close relative or friend, moving house, the breakdown of a relationship etc. Ambient stress describes that stress generated through ordinary day-to-day activities; e.g., doing the shopping, managing finances, keeping on top of daily activities such as cooking and cleaning, etc.

Discussing this model with patients can be a great aid to the development of a therapeutic alliance. It can help the patient to develop an understanding of why this has happened to them and to feel less isolated and more normal. Kingdon and Turkington (1996) argue that patients often draw catastrophic conclusions about their diagnosis such as 'I'm mad' or 'I will be locked up', which often result in anxiety, depression and hopelessness. To counter this they recommend the use of a 'normalising rationale' which involves discussion in detail of the stress vulnerability model with the patient to explain symptoms.

It may help to explain that a number of studies have demonstrated that certain types of stress can induce psychotic symptoms in people not thought to have a predisposition to psychosis. For example, sleep deprivation can lead to visual and auditory hallucinations and paranoid ideation (Oswald, 1974). Sensory deprivation (Slade and Bentall, 1988), post-traumatic stress disorder (PTSD) (Wilcox et al., 1991), hostage situations (Siegel, 1984), solitary confinement (Grassian, 1993) and sexual abuse (Ensink, 1992) have all been found to produce psychotic phenomena. In the vast majority of cases these symptoms are transitory; that is, they disappear as soon as a normal sleep pattern is restored or normal sensory stimuli is resumed.

Sexual abuse and PTSD are slightly different and there are clearly other issues to be addressed if all the symptoms are to be reduced. Informing the patient of these studies can often be reassuring; many patients, for example, will report that they experience difficulty in sleeping or periods of prolonged isolation prior to the onset of psychotic symptoms. Kingdon and Turkington (1996) state that the aim of this approach is to lead the patient 'to an understanding that there is probably a discernible reason or reasons why the symptoms have occurred and the possibility that anyone stressed in certain ways could become psychotic' (p. 106).

This normalising rationale is not only of use to patients but may be of great value to other professionals and members of the public. Emerson (1992) states that one of the main themes providing a base to normalisation is that of role expectancy. He argues that the way society reacts towards a person with a label such as mental illness often determines the behaviour and characteristics of that person. For example, a person with a diagnosis of schizophrenia may be less likely to succeed in gaining employment, and repeated failures at job seeking may convince the person that they are not capable of working. O'Brien and Tyne (1981) have described this as 'vicious circles'. Mental health services and professionals have been shown to interpret a person's behaviour differently because of any label applied to them. This was highlighted in a study by Rosenhan (1975) who found that once a person becomes labelled as mentally ill everyday behaviours such as diary writing can be interpreted as confirmation of that label. In this case keeping a diary was described as 'obsessive writing behaviour' by nursing staff.

A normalising rationale and the stress vulnerability model are important in acute settings for two reasons. First, normalising a person's experience will help to develop the therapeutic nursing relationship. Engagement and rapport building are the essential first steps when working with people with serious mental illness and are profoundly difficult (Drury, 2000). Chadwick and Birchwood (1996) have suggested some factors which may prevent engagement with clients who are experiencing serious mental illness. They include, amongst others, the patient's view of the effects of discussing their symptoms (for example, does this prevent discharge from hospital or result in an increase in medication) and an inability on the part of the nurse to empathise with the patient's experience of their symptoms because the symptoms are outside the realm of the nurse's experience. Work by Tien (1991) demonstrated that 2.3% of the normal general population experience auditory hallucinations, and discussing this with patients is extremely useful.

Many people can recall a time when they have experienced some type of psychotic phenomena (hearing their name called when they are very tired, for example) and any personal disclosure of this nature may be helpful, especially focusing on any feelings or anxiety experienced. However, it is not necessary to have experienced psychosis in order to understand how frightening the consequences might be; i.e., it is not necessary to have experienced a thought that someone is trying to kill you to understand that this thought, if you believed it, would be very frightening.

Second, it is important to consider the stress vulnerability model when one considers the environment of an acute in-patient ward. The model assumes that in psychosis, stress in the environment interacts with a person's genetic vulnerability resulting in the production of, or an increase in, symptoms of psychosis. It is generally accepted that acute wards are stressful places in which to work, often resulting in low morale and high levels of staff sickness. If working on these wards is stressful for staff, consider the impacts for patients who have an illness known to react unfavourably to stress.

Many acute wards experience high levels of patient anger and aggression and it is often assumed that this violence is due to underlying pathology. However, is this really the case? We know from the document *Safer Services* (Appleby, 1999) that people with a serious mental illness are more likely to harm themselves rather than others so why is there so much aggression in in-patient areas? One theory of aggression, the frustration theory, first described by Dollard et al. (1939) and later by Buss (1966) and Rix (1985), suggests that aggression occurs due to a build-up of frustration which the person can only release through aggression. This theory is often in keeping with an individual's own ideas of aggression; the majority of people can recall a time when they became aggressive (verbally or physically) as a response to increasing frustration or stress.

It is easy to see when admission to a psychiatric ward, often against your will, can result in a build-up of frustration in some patients. Couple this with the amount of anxiety provoking psychotic symptoms the person is experiencing due to their relapse and then add the implications of the stress vulnerability model suggesting that an increase in stress leads to an increase in symptoms. Perhaps this model offers some explanation for the levels of patient anger and aggression. There are, of course, other risk factors to be considered such as past history and presence of threat control override symptoms.

How does this hypothesis help the nurse to reduce the level of assaults in acute settings? There is evidence to suggest that only a very small number of assaults occur without any changes in the person's behavioural pattern, which could have been used to predict the assault (Sheridan et al., 1990). Nurses need to be aware of these changes, which include motor restlessness, pacing, agitation, pressure of speech, difficulty in concentration and appearing distracted that indicate that stress levels are increasing in patients and consider ways of helping the patient manage their stress levels more effectively (Wright, 1989).

Early intervention and early identification of relapse

Research suggests that young people may experience psychotic symptoms for a surprisingly long time before they receive their first effective treatment (Birchwood et al., 2000). Long delays in initiating treatments are associated with treatment resistance (Loebel et al., 1992), increased rates of relapse (Crow et al., 1986; Johnstone et al., 1990) and poorer social functioning (Birchwood et al., 2000). The aim of early intervention is to ensure that young people experiencing the first symptoms of psychosis receive effective help as quickly as possible and so improve their long-term prognosis. Birchwood, Fowler and Jackson (2000) suggest that the early stage of psychosis, lasting the first three or five years, is a critical period, which presents ideal opportunities for 'secondary prevention to limit or prevent disability and distress.' They argue that people in the early stages of psychosis should receive intensive treatment to prevent any deterioration.

The Initiative to Reduce the Impact of Schizophrenia (IRIS) have produced a set of guidelines which they state should 'be embraced if this radical approach to the treatment of severe mental illness is to be realised.' (Macmillan and Shiers, 2000). The guidelines highlight the need for a youth focus, an emphasis on social care and argue that care should be provided in the least restrictive setting possible. They advocate the use of low-dose neuroleptics to encourage compliance and minimise the risk of side-effects. All of these guidelines can be applied in acute in-patient settings.

Harrow et al. (1995) suggest that treatment resistance has its origins in the critical period covering the first three to five years. Birchwood et al. (2000) agree and argue that efforts should be made to focus on treatment resistance early on in the course of the illness. They suggest that cognitive therapy is useful in the acute phase of the illness to address residual symptoms. (See the following section.)

The families of young people experiencing their first episode of psychosis are of particular importance. Kuipers and Raune (2000) suggest that the impact on families caring for young people who are developing psychosis cannot be minimised. They state that there is evidence to suggest these families react in the same way and experience the same levels of stress and burden as long-term carers. (See the 'Family work' section.)

Relapse planning aims to help patients and their families detect relapses early. Knowledge that relapses can, in many cases, be identified in the very early stages, perhaps preventing the need for hospital admission, is often encouraging for both families and patients. In a study of depression in schizophrenia, Birchwood et al. (1992) found that a lack of perceived control over illness was linked closely with the presence of depression.

McCandless-Glincher et al. (1986), in a study of 62 patients, found that the majority of patients are able to identify a period of reduced well-being prior to relapse. Relapse planning involves teaching the patient to identify the symptoms that indicated that they are becoming unwell and developing coping strategies to prevent further relapse. Birchwood (1996) suggests that it is useful to think of these symptoms as a relapse signature that is individual to each patient. Just as the course of schizophrenia is different for each person with the illness, then so are the early warning signs of the relapse. Establishing these signs involves asking the patient to try and remember their last relapse and identify what changes they noticed and in what order. Use of prompt cards may be an aid to this process. Nurses working in acute in-patient settings are in the unique position to try and identify with patients and relatives any early warning signs of relapse whilst the information is still fresh in their minds. The signs (for example, spending too much money or not attending to personal hygiene) are first identified and then placed in an approximate order of what happens first. It is often useful to group the signs into three categories: early, middle and late warning signs. A collaborative action plan should then be developed in conjunction with the client, their carer and the multidisciplinary team. The plan should clearly state what action should be taken and by whom when a warning sign is observed. For example, an early warning sign might be increased irritability. This might be observed by the client or carer who would agree to inform the care coordinator, who might in turn agree to increase visits or other support. All members of the plan would agree to monitor for other signs of relapse. If further signs are observed, further action such as increased medication, reinstating coping strategies or home treatment options would be required. It is vitally important that all members of the team, especially the patient, are involved in the development of an action plan. Early signs monitoring and relapse prevention are wholly dependent on effective, collaborative working relationships between clients, carers and all involved in their care.

Individual cognitive behavioural interventions for psychosis

There is growing evidence for the efficacy for the use of cognitive behavioural techniques for psychotic symptoms (Haddock et al., 1998). Although much of this research has taken place with chronic, drug-resistant symptoms there is an increasing amount of interest in applying these techniques to acutely ill patients. Drury (2000) found that cognitive behaviour therapy (CBT) significantly reduced levels of positive symptoms and reduced days spent in hospital when offered to patients experiencing an acute episode of illness compared with a standard control group.

Cognitive behavioural techniques are based upon the link between thoughts, feelings and behaviours. That is, it is the way that we interpret an event that dictates the way that we feel about the event and what we do as a response to the event. For example, if a person is lying in bed at night and hears the gate creak there are a number of explanations or interpretations that could be made. One explanation is that it was just the wind making the gate creak in which case that person would probably feel relaxed and go back to sleep. Conversely, another person could think that the gate is creaking because someone is outside the house and trying to break in; this person is liable to feel very anxious and may call the police or get up to look outside. It is proposed that the interpretations a person makes are influenced by their mood, their past experiences or their beliefs.

In the example above, a person may be more likely to believe their house was being burgled if they had heard about robberies in the area or if they believe that robberies are a common event. Interpretations are then reinforced by the way a person interprets any new information. For example, suppose the person in the example above got up and looked out of the window and saw the gate open and knocking against the post. The first person would believe that they were right and it was the just the wind, whereas the second person could believe that the gate was open because the intruder had left it like that and run away. Both would have their beliefs confirmed. It is vital to human survival that we are able to interpret events quickly without much conscious thought. Imagine crossing a busy road when a car comes quickly towards you; you do not have time to weigh up the likely outcomes and must react instantly to get out of the way. The mind interprets the event as dangerous and reacts accordingly to the perceived threat. In psychosis it is hypothesised that the onset of the psychosis produces physiological changes in the brain which are then interpreted as threatening. The brain seeks out an explanation or interpretation of the threat (Nelson, 1997). As discussed above, the interpretation will usually be influenced by the person's mood, past experiences or beliefs. For example, it is only likely that an individual who had some knowledge or belief about the existence of aliens would develop an explanation revolving around aliens for what is happening to them. It is important to remember that the development of explanations or interpretations is not completed at a conscious level. This explanation is then reinforced in the same way as all other non-psychotic explanations or beliefs are reinforced; new information will be interpreted to fit it with the existing belief.

Cognitive behavioural interventions for psychosis tend to follow the same overall structure of assessment, devising a problem list, discussion of a shared model of the problem(s), the development of an individual case formulation, symptom-focused intervention, schema-focused interventions and ending with relapse prevention (Morrison, 1998). Whilst it may not be possible to complete all aspects of these interventions whilst a person is an in-patient, this structure does provide a useful direction to nurses and other professionals working in in-patient areas.

Problem list and assessment

Patients who are admitted to acute in-patient wards are liable to have diverse and complex needs; therefore, a thorough assessment of a range of potential problem areas is required. A useful start to this process is to collaboratively establish a problem list with the patient. This list should contain not only those problems identified by the patient but also those identified by the professional such as risk issues and the need to maintain social inclusion. The problems should be taken from the patient's perspective of what is happening to them. For example, for a patient who is experiencing a delusional belief that he is the son of God may not see this as a problem, but it may be a problem to him that others do not believe him and he becomes angry and aggressive as a result of the others' doubt. The problem would therefore be that X becomes angry and aggressive when others doubt him. As it is not possible to change the reactions of others, the aim would be to help the client cope more appropriately.

The remainder of this section will focus on the assessment of symptoms. The assessment process should aim to establish what symptoms are present and then compile a detailed description of each symptom. The professional should start by attempting to establish the basic components of the problem/symptom by obtaining answers to the following: What is the problem? When does the problem occur? Where does the problem occur? Who is the problem better or worse with? Why does the problem occur; that is, what is the feared consequence of the problem? This sequence of questions is often referred to as the five Ws of assessment. It is important to remember that the five Ws refer to the information required, not the actual question. Therefore, when attempting to establish what part of the sequence, the nurse might ask, 'can you tell me something about the events which led up to your admission to hospital?' Following on from this information it is important to next establish the frequency, intensity and duration of the symptom. This information will provide a helpful baseline with which to monitor the effectiveness of any intervention. Finally a three-system analysis of each symptom should be completed. The aim is to establish the person's thoughts, feelings and behaviours before the occurrence of the symptom, during occurrence and afterwards. It will usually take several sessions with the person to establish all of these aspects. It will be helpful to ask the person to complete a diary of the occurrence of the particular symptom that includes columns for the person to record what they were thinking, feeling and doing before, during and after the symptom has occurred. For most patients in the acute stage of their illness, this task is too complex and it will be more helpful to ask the patient to record only the presence (frequency) of their symptom in the first instance, moving on to more detailed recordings over time.

The use of structured assessment tools will help to provide further information. Global tools such the PANSS (Positive and Negative Symptom Scale) (Kay et al., 1989) will help to identify symptoms, and more specific scales such as the Psychotic Symptom Ratings Scales (PSYRATS) (Haddock et al., 1998) and Belief About Voices Questionnaire (BAVQ) (Chadwick and Birchwood, 1996) will be useful to clarify the differing dimensions of each symptom.

Case formulation

The use of a normalising rationale, as discussed earlier, should be used with patients not only as an aid to the development of a therapeutic relationship but also as a way of developing a shared understanding of what is happening to them. This represents the beginnings of a case formulation; for further discussion of case formulation in psychosis see Haddock and Tarrier (2000) and Morrison (1998).

Symptom-focused interventions

The development of symptom-focused coping strategies is of particular relevance to an acute in-patient setting. As previously stated, patients are usually admitted to acute settings when they are extremely ill and experiencing high stress. Effective problem solving is hindered greatly at times of high stress and so it is usual that people are not able to implement their own effective coping strategies as well as at other times. If you consider stressful periods in your own life it is not unusual to recall increased irritability or anger or increased use of alcohol or smoking.

A beneficial approach to helping patients develop more effective coping strategies is coping strategy enhancement (Tarrier et al., 1993; Yusopoff and Tarrier, 1996). This approach begins with a detailed assessment of the patient's current coping strategies. The person is asked to record what coping strategies they use and to rate their effectiveness. No value judgements are made regarding the coping strategies but the positive and negative effects of each strategy are discussed. New coping strategies are then introduced and the patient will be asked to try them and rate their effectiveness. The strategy should be explained during the session and the person will need the opportunity to practice before attempting to use the strategy when the symptoms occur. A helpful way to do this is to ask the person to imagine the occurrence of the problematic symptom and then practise the new coping strategy. New strategies should be introduced one at a time. The following session should consider the effectiveness of the new strategy and its positive and negative effects. Further new strategies should be introduced until the patient has a variety of methods to help them cope with their symptoms. Finally, a process of activity scheduling is used to help the patient incorporate their new coping strategies into their daily life. For example, during the assessment process it was discovered that X was more likely to experience auditory hallucinations when in crowded places such as the supermarket. It is found that a useful coping strategy for X is sub-vocalisation. Sub-vocalisation is based upon the premise that auditory hallucinations are misattributed internal thoughts. The generation of internal thoughts involves the use of the muscles of the vocal cords in a similar way to speech.

The theory suggests that auditory hallucinations can be blocked if the muscles involved in their occurrence (i.e., the muscles of the vocal cords) are used in another way either by speaking or by concentrating on something else and generating other internal thoughts. It may not always be possible for X to go and speak to someone when his voices occur and so the activity scheduling would suggest the most appropriate and available strategy for the setting. For example, when X is in the supermarket the most appropriate strategy might be to take a shopping list and read the list when he feels himself becoming anxious or begins to hear the voices. Other useful coping strategies to suggest are those which help patients effectively manage stress levels and anxiety associated with the symptoms or diagnosis. These would include relaxation techniques, positive self-talk and other distraction techniques.

The use of coping strategy enhancement is dependent upon the motivation of the patient and so a clear rationale for the intervention should be given. This rationale should focus on the value of increasing one's ways of dealing with a problem but not make any value judgements regarding the patient's current ways of coping.

Family work

The interest in the importance of families was generated by Brown and his colleagues at the Social Psychiatry Unit, London, in the 1950s. They investigated the circumstances of patients with schizophrenia who were discharged home to live with parents as opposed to those who went to live alone or in hostels. Surprisingly, they found that living alone was more favourable for patients, in terms of levels of relapse, than living with family members. To investigate this further, Brown and his colleagues hypothesised that there was something happening in the family environment that was responsible for the relapses. From this hypothesis, the concept of expressed emotion (EE) was born. To measure this, an interview schedule entitled the Camberwell Family Interview (CFI) was developed to interview patients' families (Leff et al., 1985). The CFI measures five components of EE: amount of critical remarks, hostility, emotional over-involvement, warmth and positive remarks. However, in practice only the three negative measures (critical remarks, hostility and emotional over-involvement) are predictive of relapse (Vaughn and Leff, 1976). Leff et al. (1985) continued the work of Brown and further developed the scale. They found that the amount of face-to-face contact that the patient has with their family was important, over 35 hours per week being considered high, as was the patient's compliance (or not) with their medication. They found that the biggest predictor of relapse involved the following combination of risk factors: spending more than 35 hours per week in direct contact with a relative who has high expressed emotion and not adhering with medication regimes; over 90% of this group relapsed within 9 months (Leff et al., 1985).

Various studies have tried to establish why there is this apparent interaction between high expressed emotion, high face-to-face contact and relapse. Barrowclough and Tarrier (1992) reviewed these studies and suggest that the levels of arousal within the sympathetic nervous system of patients with schizophrenia are increased when they are with a high EE relative and this response is maintained with high levels of face-to-face contact. They suggest that 'this physiological reaction is in response to the stress of living with a relative who is critical, hostile and emotionally over-involved'. These levels of stress accumulate and interact with the patient's own vulnerability to produce the symptoms of schizophrenia, and therefore the relapse.

Family interventions are based on the hypothesis that if there is a link between high expressed emotions in relatives and relapse of patients with schizophrenia then any intervention aimed at reducing the levels of expressed emotion in the relative could help to prevent relapse in the patient. Various studies have investigated this hypothesis and have, on the whole, reduced relapse rates quite substantially. The Camberwell study by Leff et al. (1985) compared family therapy, which consisted of an education programme regarding schizophrenia for relatives, a relatives group and individual family therapy, plus standard NHS care with standard care alone. Following 9 months of intervention, relapse rates were 8% in the family intervention group compared to 50% in the control group. At 2 years follow-up the relapse rates were 20% in the family intervention group and 78% in the control group. This demonstrates that the effects do, at least in part, last beyond the course of the therapy.

Falloon (1985) offered family therapy or supportive psychotherapy to 36 patients with schizophrenia and their families. The family therapy consisted of education, communication skills training and training in problem-solving techniques. In the first 9 months of treatment each group received 25 sessions. After nine months, sessions were held once a month for two years. At the end of the intervention, the relapse rates were 6% for the family therapy group and 44% for the supportive psychotherapy group. This study demonstrates the superiority of family intervention in reducing relapse rates when compared to supportive psychotherapy.

These two studies demonstrate that family interventions are successful at reducing relapse rates but it is important to consider which parts of the family intervention package are the most useful. A study in Hamburg (Dulz and Hand, 1986) offered group analytical psychotherapy to patients and their high EE relatives, a 'no treatment' group was used as a control. The patients and relatives received the therapy separately. The differences in the relapse rates were not as substantial in this study as in other studies; i.e., 36% for the treatment group and 54% for the control group. It has been suggested that this is because analytical treatments are in themselves stressful and may have caused some relapses (Strachan et al., 1986).

To try and establish which components of family therapy are useful, Tarrier et al. (1989) compared family intervention which included education, stress management and goal planning, with education alone for a second group and routine treatment for the third. Groups 1 and 2 also received routine treatment. The relapse rates were 12% for the family intervention group, 43% for the education group and 53% for standard treatment alone. This would suggest that education packages (when offered without family therapy) are not useful in reducing relapse rates. However, most authors would agree that education is an essential component of family therapy and is useful to help the families understand the importance of stress and the stress vulnerability model of psychosis (Barrowclough and Tarrier, 1992).

This research is important in an acute setting for a number of reasons. First, the ideal time to engage with families for family intervention has been found to be whilst the person is experiencing an acute episode of the illness (Hudson, 1975). During this time the family are likely to be experiencing high levels of stress and concern for their relative and willing to engage in any new treatment that may prevent this relapse from happening again. Families may be feeling partly or totally responsible for the relapse at this point in time and so it is essential to consider how to phrase the rationale for family interventions to the family. Discussions of expressed emotion, however well intended or phrased, are not helpful. Many families are aware of the family interaction theories which, despite little, if any, evidence, proposed that families (especially mothers) are responsible for causing schizophrenia. Barrowclough and Tarrier (1992) suggest that it is useful to view the families as 'rehabilitative agents' that is an important factor in maintaining the mental well-being of patients. A rationale for family work should acknowledge the importance of the work families do as carers and how services would not succeed in caring for the seriously mentally ill without this input from families. Take time for a second to imagine how services would cope (if at all) if no family members took on any caring role. Another important aspect to consider, when discussing the rationale for family intervention, is that these families are reacting in normal ways to abnormal situations. It is normal to experience anxiety and stress when faced with difficult situations. For example, common symptoms of schizophrenia, negative symptoms which can be described as the 'absence of normal functioning' (Hogg, 1996) (e.g., speech impairment, under-activity and loss of interest and pleasure in things) can be incredibly frustrating for relatives. Imagine how you would feel if your son has no motivation to do anything, does not appear to enjoy anything and you do not know why.

However, it should not be taken that lack of knowledge is the reason that this situation is found to be stressful. Moore et al. (1992) found that caring for patients with negative symptoms frequently provokes criticisms from staff and is one area of work that staff find incredibly frustrating.

It should be remembered that serious mental illness is not unique in its ability to invoke stress and anxiety in the relatives of sufferers. Most people will be able to identify increasing levels of stress when a family member has been ill. This stress may manifest itself in a variety of ways, which will include becoming emotionally over-involved with the person or feeling irritable and hostile.

Importance of assessment, psycho-education

Whilst it may not be possible to offer a full package of family interventions, which require at least nine months of intervention, to patients and their families in an acute in-patient setting, it is possible to adapt the model of intervention. The families (with the patient's consent) should be involved at every stage of their relatives' care. They will be able to provide a wealth of information regarding the patient and this current relapse. This will be particularly helpful when trying to establish any changes in the patient's behaviour which preceded this relapse and so help to identify a relapse signature.

Presenting a rationale to the families for family intervention as discussed above is also very useful. Nurses should attempt to emphasise to the family the importance of their role as carers and normalise any feelings of stress the family is experiencing. As highlighted above, whilst educating the family about schizophrenia may in itself not prevent relapse, it has been found useful to help with the relatives' levels of burden, distress and anxiety.

Barrowclough and Tarrier (1992) also suggest that education is a useful way of engaging the family members to more long-term interventions. They suggest that it is useful to adopt an interactive model of education when working with families. That is to firstly describe the common features of schizophrenia and then help the families to adapt this knowledge to their actual experience of their relative's illness. They state that relatives may have already formed opinions of why various symptoms occur and, for example, may agree that delusions are a symptom of schizophrenia but will still believe that their son or daughter is living in fantasy land or being stupid when he or she expresses their delusional ideation.

This education can be completed by first giving the relatives information about general symptomatology (leaflets may be a useful way of doing this) and then giving specific information relating to the patient's own symptoms. This education package can then be reinforced every time the staff member speaks to the relative. For example, in the case of delusional ideas it would be first necessary to describe delusions as a symptom of schizophrenia, then individualise the education to describe the family members' belief that he or she is related to royalty, for example, as a delusion. This can then be reinforced throughout treatment. For example, one would describe delusional ideas as odd or bizarre beliefs, held by the person with some level of conviction, that are not in keeping with the person's culture and then state, for example, when X tells you that he or she is related to royalty this is a symptom of their illness. It would be useful at this point to establish how the relative feels they cope with this symptom and advice can be given on various appropriate responses, such as a response that would neither collude with nor dismiss the delusion. Families often report that they do not know what to say or do for the best when certain symptoms are present and greatly value any constructive advice.

The education package should emphasise the importance of stress and its negative consequences, both for the patient and the relative. This would then lead on to advice regarding stress management techniques. Again it is important to normalise the occurrence of stress within family members when a relative is ill to ensure that no blame is construed. The rationale for stress management is often best phrased in terms of caring for the carers. The stress is usually experienced as a response to the patient's behaviour; therefore, it is possible to address this problem through two routes: the behaviour of the patient or the response of the relative.

Stabilising symptoms and lessening troublesome behaviours is one of the foremost aims of an acute ward and so indirectly this should help the relative. Owing to time restrictions, it may not be possible to help the patient's relatives to reframe their negative cognitions associated with the patient's behaviours whilst the patient is an in-patient, but it will be possible to offer advice regarding general stress reduction techniques and coping mechanisms. This might include relaxation and encouraging the relative to spend more time enjoying their own interests. This latter intervention may have the added benefit of helping to reduce the amount of face-to-face contact the patient has with their relatives.

Conclusion

This chapter has described the importance of psychosocial interventions and has discussed their relevance in in-patient settings. Psychosocial interventions are evidence-based interventions, which have been shown to have greatly beneficial effects for clients. This statement alone should emphasise the need to implement these interventions in the acute in-patient settings where the patients are usually demonstrating the highest level of complexity and need. Much has been written regarding the difficulties of working within these areas often due to staff shortages, high bed occupancy and complexity of patient need, and these difficulties are sometimes suggested as a reason that psychosocial interventions are not wholesale practice within these areas. However, the writers argue that the implementation of the philosophy of psychosocial interventions could easily be achieved. These interventions are based upon the stress vulnerability model of psychosis; that is, that increasing stress levels result in increasing symptoms and strategies which help the patient to manage their stress more effectively and will help to control symptoms. The interventions are structured following a process of assessment, formulation, intervention and evaluation and are collaborative aiming to work from the person's subjective view of what is happening to them. It is of little importance that a person may be experiencing a delusional belief as the majority of people hold idiosyncratic beliefs based on little evidence; what is important is the distress or problems caused to the person or others as a result of that belief. Surely it is not unreasonable to suggest that in-patient areas can easily implement interventions which are based upon a structure that involves including the patient in all aspects of their care and aims to help that person cope effectively with any stressors in their environment. If this can be achieved then the implementation of psychosocial interventions is well under way.

References

Appleby, L. (1999) *Safer Services: National Confidential Inquiry into Suicide and Homicide by People with Mental Illness.* London: Department of Health.

Baguley, I. and Baguley, C. (1999) 'Psychosocial interventions in the treatment of psychosis', *Mental Health Care*, 2 (9): 314–16.

Barrowclough, C. and Tarrier, N. (1992) *Families of Schizophrenic Patients*. Cheltenham: Thornes.

Bateson, G., Jackson, D., Haley, J. and Weakland, J. (1956) 'Towards a theory of schizophrenia', *Behavioural Science*, 1: 251–64.

Birchwood, M. (1996) 'Early intervention in psychotic relapse: cognitive approaches to detection and management', in G. Haddock and P.D. Slade (eds), *Cognitive–Behavioural Interventions with Psychotic Disorders*. London: Routledge.

Birchwood, M., Fowler, D. and Jackson, C. (2000) 'Preface', in *Early Intervention in Psychosis*. Chichester: Wiley.

Birchwood, M., Smith, J. and Cochrane, R. (1992) 'Specific and non-specific effects of educational intervention for families living with schizophrenia: a comparison of three methods', *British Journal of Psychiatry*, 160: 806–14.

Brown, G.W. (1959) 'Experiences of discharged chronic mental hospital patients in various types of living group', *Millbank Memorial Fund Quarterly*, 37: 105–31.

Brown, G.W., Carstairs, G.M. and Topping, G. (1958) 'Post hospital adjustment of chronic mental patients', *Lancet,* ii: 685–9.

Buss, A.H. (1966) 'The effect of harm on subsequent aggression', *Journal of Experimental Research in Personality*, 3: 249–55.

Chadwick, P. and Birchwood, M. (1996) 'Cognitive therapy for voices', in G. Haddock and P.D. Slade (eds), *Cognitive–Behavioural Interventions with Psychotic Disorders*. London: Routledge.

Crow, T.J., MacMillan, J.F., Johnson, A.L. et al. (1986) 'II: A randomised controlled trial of prophylactic neuroleptic treatment', *British Journal of Psychiatry*, 159: 790–4.

Department of Health (2002) *Mental Health Policy Implementation Guide: Adult Acute Inpatient Care Provision*. London: Department of Health.

Dollard, J., Doob, L., Miller, N., Mowrer, O. and Sears, R. (1939) *Frustration and Aggression*. New Haven, CT: Yale University Press.

Drury, V. (2000) 'Cognitive therapy in early psychosis', in M. Birchwood, D. Fowler and C. Jackson (eds), *Early Intervention in Psychosis*. Chichester: Wiley.

Dulz, B. and Hand, I. (1986) 'Short term relapse in young schizophrenics. Can it be predicted and affected by family (CFI), patient and treatment variables? An experimental study', in M.J. Goldstein, I. Hand and K. Halweg (eds), *The Treatment of Schizophrenia: Family Assessment and Intervention*. Berlin: Springer-Verlag.

Emerson, E. (1992) 'What is normalisation?', in H. Brown and H. Smith (eds), *Normalisation: A Reader for the Nineties*. London: Routledge.

Ensink, B.J. (1992) *Confusing Realities: A Study on Child Sexual Abuse and Psychiatric Symptoms*. Amsterdam: Free University Press.

Falloon, R.H. (1985) *Family Management of Schizophrenia: A Study of Clinical, Social, Family and Economic Benefits*. Baltimore, MD: Johns Hopkins University Press.

Grassian, G. (1993) 'Psychopathology of solitary confinement', *American Journal of Psychiatry*, 140: 1450–4.

Haddock, G. and Tarrier, N. (2000) 'Assessment and formulation in the cognitive behavioural treatment of psychosis', in N. Tarrier, A. Wells and G. Haddock (eds), *Treating Complex Cases: The Cognitive Behavioural Approach*. Chichester: Wiley.

Haddock, G., McCarron, J., Tarrier, N. and Faragher, E.B. (1998) 'Scales to measure dimensions of delusions and hallucinations: the Psychotic Symptom Ratings Scales (PSYRATS)', *Psychological Medicine*, 29 (4): 879–89.

Harrow, M., MacDonald, A.W., Sands, J.R. and Silverstein, M.L. (1995) 'Vulnerability to delusions over time in schizophrenia and affective disorders', *Schizophrenia Bulletin*, 21: 95–109.

Hogg, L. (1996) 'Psychological treatments for negative symptoms', in G. Haddock and P.D. Slade (eds), *Cognitive–Behavioural Interventions with Psychotic Disorders.* London: Routledge.

Hudson, B. (1975) 'A behaviour modification project with chronic schizophrenics in the community', *Behaviour Research and Therapy*, 13: 339–41.

Johnstone, E.C., MacMillan, J.F., Frith, C.D., Benn, D.K. and Crow, T.J. (1990) 'Further investigation of the predictors of outcome following first schizophrenic episodes', *British Journal of Psychiatry*, 157: 182–9.

Kay, S.R., Opler, L.A. and Lindenmayer, J.P. (1989) 'The Positive and Negative Symptom Scale (PANSS) rationale and standardisation', *British Journal of Psychiatry*, 155 (Supplement 7): 59–65.

Kingdon, D.G. and Turkington, D. (1996) 'Using a normalising rationale in the treatment of schizophrenic patients', in G. Haddock and P.D. Slade (eds), *Cognitive–Behavioural Interventions with Psychotic Disorders.* London: Routledge.

Kuipers, E. and Raune, D. (2000) 'The early development of expressed emotion and burden in the families of first onset psychosis', in M. Birchwood, D. Fowler and C. Jackson (eds), *Early Intervention in Psychosis.* Chichester: Wiley.

Lancashire, S., Haddock, G., Butterworth, T., Tarrier, N. and Baguley, I. (1996) 'Training mental health professionals to use psychosocial interventions with people who have severe mental health problems', *Clinician*, 14 (1): 32–40.

Leff, J.P. and Vaughn, C. (1980) 'The integration of life events and relatives' expressed emotion in schizophrenia and depressive neurosis', *British Journal of Psychiatry*, 36: 146–53.

Leff, J., Kuipers, L., Berowitz, R. and Sturgeon, D. (1985) 'A controlled trial of social intervention in the families of schizophrenic patients: 2 year follow up', *British Journal of Psychiatry*, 146: 594–600.

Lidz, T., Cornelissen, A., Fleck, S. and Terry, D. (1957) 'The intrafamilial environment of schizophrenic patients: II. Marital schism and marital skew', *American Journal of Psychiatry*, 114: 241–8.

Loebel, A.D., Lieberman, J.A., Avir, J.M.J. et al. (1992) 'Duration of psychosis and outcome in first episode schizophrenia', *American Journal of Psychiatry*, 149: 1183–8.

McCandless-Glincher, L., McKnight, S., Hamera, E., Smith, B.L., Peterson, K. and Plumelee, A.A. (1986) 'Use of symptoms by schizophrenics to monitor and regulate their illness', *Hospital and Community Psychiatry*, 37: 929–33.

Macmillan, F. and Shiers, D. (2000) 'The IRIS programme', in M. Birchwood, D. Fowler and C. Jackson (eds), *Early Intervention in Psychosis: A Guide to Concepts, Evidence and Interventions.* Chichester: Wiley.

MHAC/SCMH (Mental Health Act Commission/Sainsbury Centre for Mental Health) (1997) *The National Visit: A One-day Visit to 309 Acute Psychiatric Wards.* London: Sainsbury Centre for Mental Health.

Moore, E., Ball, R.A. and Kuipers, L. (1992) 'Expressed emotion in staff working with the long term mentally ill', *British Journal of Psychiatry*, 161: 802–8.

Morrison, A.P. (1998) 'Cognitive behaviour therapy for psychotic symptoms in schizophrenia', in N. Tarrier, A. Wells and G. Haddock (eds), *Treating Complex Cases: The Cognitive Behavioural Therapy Approach.* Chichester: Wiley.

Nelson, H. (1997) *Cognitive Behavioural Therapy with Schizophrenia: A Practice Manual.* Cheltenham: Thornes.

O'Brien, J. and Tyne, A. (1981) *The Principle of Normalisation: A Foundation for Effective Services.* London: Values into Action.

Oswald, I. (1974) *Sleep*, 3rd edn. Harmondsworth: Penguin.

Rix, G. (1985) 'Compassion is better than conflict', *Nursing Times*, 81 (38): 18–24.

Rosenhan, D.L. (1975) 'On being sane in insane places', in T. Scheff (ed.), *Labelling Madness*. Englewood Cliffs, NJ: Prentice Hall.

Sainsbury Centre for Mental Health (SCMH) (1998) *Acute Problems: A Survey of the Quality of Care in Acute Psychiatric Wards*. London: Sainsbury Centre for Mental Health.

Sheridan, M., Henrion, R., Robinson, L. and Baxter, V. (1990) 'Precipitants of violence in a psychiatric setting', *Hospital and Community Psychiatry*, 41: 776–80.

Siegel, R.K. (1984) 'Hostage hallucinations', *Journal of Nervous and Mental Disease*, 172: 264–71.

Slade, P. and Bentall, R. (1988) *Sensory Deception: A Scientific Analysis of Hallucination*. London: Croom Helm.

Strachan, A.M., Leff, J.P., Goldstein, M.J., Doane, J.A. and Burtt, C. (1986) 'Emotion attitudes and direct communication in the families of schizophrenics: a cross national replication', *British Journal of Psychiatry*, 149: 279–87.

Tarrier, N., Barrowclough, C., Vaughn, C. et al. (1989) 'The community management of schizophrenia: a two year follow up of a behavioural intervention with families', *British Journal of Psychiatry*, 154: 625–8.

Tarrier, N., Beckett, R., Harwood, S., Baker, A., Yusopoff, L. and Ugarteburu, I. (1993) 'A trial of two cognitive behavioural methods of treating drug resistant residual psychotic symptoms in schizophrenic patients. I. Outcome', *British Journal of Psychiatry*, 162: 524–32.

Tien, A.Y. (1991) 'Distribution of hallucinations in the population', *Social Psychiatry and Psychiatric Epidemiology*, 26: 287–92.

Vaughn, C.E. and Leff, J.P. (1976) 'The influence of family and social factors on the course of psychiatric illness', *British Journal of Psychiatry*, 129: 125–37.

Vaughn, C.E. and Leff, J.P. (1981) 'Patterns of emotional response in relatives of schizophrenic patients', *Schizophrenia Bulletin*, 7: 43–4.

Wright, R. (1989) 'Threatening behaviour', *Nursing Times*, 85 (42): 26–9.

Yusopoff, L. and Tarrier, N. (1996) 'Coping strategy enhancement for persistent hallucinations and delusions', in. G. Haddock and P.D. Slade (eds), *Cognitive Behavioural Interventions with Psychotic Disorders*. London: Routledge.

Zubin, J. and Spring, B. (1977) 'Vulnerability – a new view of schizophrenia', *Journal of Abnormal Psychology*, 86: 103–26.

ELEVEN
Medication management
Richard Gray

Summary

A considerable amount of time is spent helping patients, mainly suffering from psychotic illnesses, to manage their medication. Anti-psychotic medication is without doubt effective in alleviating psychotic symptoms such as hallucinations and delusions. If taken continuously anti-psychotic medication is also effective at keeping psychotic symptoms under control (preventing relapse) allowing people to leave hospital and hopefully continue with their lives. However, anti-psychotic medication does not fulfil its clinical potential with many more people relapsing once they leave hospital than necessary. This is, at least in part, as a result of non-compliance with medication. The reasons why people stop taking their medication are complex but some of the more important factors that affect compliance include patients' awareness of their illness, their beliefs about treatment, the side-effects they experience from medication and their use of non-prescribed substances.

Evidence from clinical trials shows that medication management should consist of the following.

- A collaborative approach to working with patients.
- Use of valid and reliable assessment tools to measure psychopathology, anti-psychotic side-effects, attitudes towards treatment, insight and compliance.
- Logical prescribing of anti-psychotic medication.
- Effective management of anti-psychotic side-effects.
- The provision of information about illness and treatment.
- Tailoring medication regimes to suit the patient.
- Use of compliance therapy techniques.

Such practice has been shown to enhance compliance and prevent relapse, issues highlighted in *Addressing Acute Concerns* (SNMAC, 1999), which emphasises the need for mental health nurses working in acute care settings to be provided with the medication management skills they need to be able to effectively help patients manage their medication.

Background

Mental health nurses working in acute psychiatry spend a substantial amount of time helping patients to manage their medication. The majority of patients admitted to acute wards suffer from psychotic disorders, predominantly schizophrenia. Consequently, this chapter focuses on the management of anti-psychotic drugs used to treat their symptoms, although many of the principles apply equally to the management of medicines used in the treatment of many other conditions.

Schizophrenia

Schizophrenia is a debilitating mental disorder characterised by a range of symptoms including: delusions, formal thought disorder, hallucinations, abnormal affect, passivity phenomena, motor abnormalities, cognitive deficits, lack of volition and lack of insight (WHO, 1992). The presentation of the illness varies tremendously, not only between individuals, but within the same individual at different stages of their illness.

Until recently the course of schizophrenia was considered to be one of continuous deterioration (Shepherd et al., 1989). However, very few studies have followed people with schizophrenia beyond the middle decades of life. Long-term studies that have been carried out suggest that schizophrenia tends to have a prolonged course with the greatest variability in the initial stages (Bleuler, 1974; Ciompi, 1980), making aggressive early treatment of vital importance.

Pharmacological treatment of schizophrenia

Anti-psychotic medication has been the mainstay of treatment for schizophrenia since the 1950s when it was discovered that the dopamine antagonists haloperidol and chlorpromazine exerted anti-psychotic effects. The dopamine hypothesis of schizophrenia is supported by reports that the clinical potency of anti-psychotics is proportional to the extent to which they block dopamine receptors (Creese et al., 1976). These observations led to the widespread belief that excessive dopamine activity or hyperdopaminergia was associated with the pathophysiology of schizophrenia.

According to the dopamine hypothesis, anti-psychotic agents ameliorate the positive symptoms of schizophrenia through dopamine D_2 blockade in the mesolimbic system. In fact, *in vitro* studies have shown a linear relationship between anti-psychotic potency and D_2 blockade (Pilowsky et al., 1992). Developments in imaging techniques such as positron emission tomography (PET) and single photon emission tomography (SPET) have made it possible to carry out *in vivo* studies visualising receptor binding sites in the brain. One PET study showed that a relatively modest dose of haloperidol (2 mg/day) resulted in 53–74% occupancy of available D_2 receptors (Farde et al., 1992). This has important clinical implications as it suggests that there is a maximum effective dose, above which there is no improvement in efficacy and a possible decline in tolerability.

An inadequate response to treatment with neuroleptics may be encountered in more than 30% of patients with schizophrenia (Kane, 1989). It has been hypothesised, but not confirmed, that a poor response to anti-psychotic medication is due to inadequate occupancy of central D_2 receptors. One SPET study showed no significant difference in striatal D_2 receptor availability among anti-psychotic responders ($n = 10$), anti-psychotic non-responders ($n = 8$) and normal controls ($n = 20$) (Pilowsky et al., 1993), suggesting that a poor clinical response cannot be attributed to inadequate striatal D_2 occupancy.

Other reports suggest that a high affinity for D_2 receptors may not be the only basis for efficacy in antipsychotic agents. Although these drugs typically occupy these receptors within a few hours of administration, there is often a delay of one to three weeks before therapeutic benefits are reported (Gray, 1998a). This suggests that these drugs act via a series of secondary, and as yet unknown, processes that evolve over days to weeks. There are suggestions that a number of other neuroreceptors, peptides and amino acid systems may be involved, supported by the fact that changes in systems other than the dopamine system have been implicated in the aetiology of schizophrenia. These include: serotonin, glutamate, noradrenaline, neurotensin and aminobutyric acid.

Chlorpromazine, the first effective pharmacological treatment for the symptoms of schizophrenia, was introduced during the 1950s. Since then, a variety of anti-psychotic agents have been developed. Controlled clinical trials have repeatedly shown that these drugs are generally efficacious for the positive symptoms of schizophrenia. However, tolerability problems, especially acute extra-pyramidal symptoms (EPS; dystonias, akathisia and Parkinsonism), encountered with these so-called conventional agents has prompted further research into the development of improved novel and atypical agents.

Although EPS are typically perceived as the most troublesome side-effects associated with anti-psychotic agents, other side-effects are also encountered with their use. Anti-psychotic agents have complex receptor-binding profiles that may underlie these effects. Hyperprolactinemia, caused by dopamine blockade in the tuberoinfundibular dopamine pathway, may cause sexual dysfunction, amenorrhoea, galactorrhoea or gynacomastia. The blockade of muscarinic receptor may cause anti-cholinergic symptoms (dry mouth, blurred vision, constipation) whilst the blockade of histamine receptors may induce sedation.

Atypical anti-psychotics

Perhaps the most effective way of minimising the risk of EPS is via the use of atypical or novel anti-psychotics that, by definition, have a low propensity to induce EPS. The early 1990s saw the introduction of clozapine, the first of a new generation of anti-psychotic drugs. However, clozapine is not a new drug. When it was first introduced into Europe during the 1970s it was met with great hope. This drug overcame many of the limitations of the conventional neuroleptics in that it appeared to reduce negative symptoms, it was associated with little or no EPS, and it was effective for patients with refractory illness. However, in 1975 agranulocytosis developed in 18 of 3,200 clozapine-treated patients in Finland, and 4 of 2,900 in Switzerland (Gray, 1999). The serious nature of this side-effect led to the voluntary withdrawal of clozapine from the market. Nonetheless, the advent of clozapine marked an important advance in the treatment of schizophrenia.

In 1988, results of a multi-centre study revealed that clozapine was more effective than conventional neuroleptics for patients with treatment-resistant schizophrenia (Kane et al., 1988). A number of controlled (Claghorn et al., 1987) and uncontrolled (Matted, 1989; Meltzer et al., 1989) studies have demonstrated that clozapine is a clinically useful drug that reduces both the positive and negative symptoms of schizophrenia with a low incidence of EPS. In 1990, it was introduced in the UK with strict guidelines for haematological monitoring because of the associated risk for agranulocytosis.

Clinical experience with clozapine has also led to the development of other novel anti-psychotic agents, including risperidone, olanzapine, sertindole, quetiapine and ziprasidone. Phase III and IV clinical trials of these agents have repeatedly shown that they have placebo levels of EPS (around 7–16%; Gray, 1999). However, there is a great deal of variability in the mode of action of these drugs. For example, risperidone and ziprasidone are potent dopamine D_2 and serotonin $5\text{-}HT_{2a}$ antagonists, whilst clozapine, olanzapine and quetiapine are multi-receptor antagonists (Moore, 1999).

In practice, because of their classical affinity for dopamine D_2 receptors, risperidone and ziprasidone will, at high doses, induce EPS. The same is not true of clozapine, olanzapine and quetiapine, however, which have a much weaker affinity for D_2 receptors and as a result do not have the propensity to induce EPS at higher doses (Bigliani et al., 1998). It has been proposed, but not confirmed, that risperidone and ziprasidone have a low incidence of EPS because of serotonin–dopamine interactions in the basal ganglia. Serotonin blockade appears to reverse the effects of dopamine D_2 blockade, but only in the nigrostriatal system and not in the mesolimbic system (Kapur and Remington, 1996). Clozapine, olanzapine and quetiapine in contrast appear to have a naturally high affinity for dopamine receptors in the mesolimbic system (Bigliani et al., 1998) and consequently a low propensity to induce EPS.

There is convincing evidence for the efficacy of conventional anti-psychotics. However, they may tend to be used in higher than necessary doses and are generally poorly tolerated. There are few data to assist in the management of many of these symptoms and the treatment of acute EPS is challenging. Novel and atypical anti-psychotics are generally very well tolerated and have a low propensity to induce many of the problematic side-effects associated with conventional treatments (Gray, 1999). Guidelines have been published to guide clinicians on how to effectively use anti-psychotics and minimise side-effects (Taylor et al., 2001), although concern has been repeatedly expressed that clinicians fail to follow such guidance.

To summarize so far:

- schizophrenia is a serious mental disorder;
- anti-psychotic medication is effective at treating predominantly the positive symptoms of the illness;
- typical anti-psychotics suffer from serious side-effects including EPS that need careful treatment and management;
- atypical anti-psychotics are much better tolerated and do not cause EPS.

The problem of non-compliance

There is good evidence that in schizophrenia, the prophylactic use of anti-psychotic medication reduces the risk of relapse (Kane, 1989; Marder, 1999). However, a number of studies have demonstrated that compliance with anti-psychotic medication is generally poor and not taking medication is associated with a substantial increase in relapse rates, more frequent hospitalisations and a generally poorer outcome in people with psychotic illnesses (Gabel and Piezcker, 1985; Helgason, 1990). Kemp et al. (1997) have proposed that the so-called 'revolving door phenomenon' can be almost exclusively attributed to repeated non-compliance. Kisling (1994) has argued that if patients were completely compliant with their medication, relapse rates would fall to about 15% (currently 50% of patients relapse within a year of achieving remission). However, the assumption that poor compliance can be attributed solely to the patient's failure to do what clinicians have told them to must be juxtaposed with evidence that professionals often do not carry out their own responsibilities regarding medication. For example, Taylor et al. (2001) showed that prescriptions for anti-psychotics are often inappropriate, resulting in unwanted and unnecessary side-effects.

It has been proposed that either 'concordance' or 'adherence' should replace the use of the word 'compliance'. Concordance emphasises patient rights, the need for information and the importance of two-way communication and decision-making. However, it is clinicians' practice rather than the language that they use that is important, and it is practice that is the focus of this chapter.

How common is non-compliance?

Estimating compliance rates in people with schizophrenia has proved difficult for two reasons. First, there is no agreed definition of compliance – definitions vary from complete cessation or verbal refusal, to any significant deviation from prescription, including dosage errors or failure to attend appointments. Second, there is no valid way of measuring compliance. Rates of compliance have been measured using a number of different methods but none has proved satisfactory. These include physicians' assessment and patients' self-report, pill counts, and urine and blood assays. These methods of assessment are not always reliable. Patient self-report and physician assessment are inaccurate, both consistently overestimating compliance (Churchill, 1985). Pill counts are more reliable, but it is impossible to tell whether the patient has actually ingested the medication. Urine testing for a drug with a long half-life will tend to overestimate compliance. Since most neuroleptics have a relatively long half-life, blood assay is likely to prove more reliable. However, the degree of compliance is impossible to determine and therefore blood assays can only be used as a criterion for current compliance (Babiker, 1986).

The problem of accurately measuring adherence explains inconsistencies in the incidence of non-compliance reported in people with schizophrenia. For example, Quitkin et al. (1978) used clinician judgement to determine compliance and observed that only 10% of patients were non-compliant with their medication over a 12-month period. In contrast, Wolff and Colacino (1961), using patient interviews over a 6-month period, reported that 73% of patients were non-compliant. However, in a review of the world literature Cramer and Rosenheck (1998) proposed an average non-compliance rate of approximately 42%, a finding that is similar to rates in other mental and physical disorders.

Why are patients non-compliant?

Difficulties in reliably measuring compliance not only make it challenging to quantify the incidence but also to produce a model to explain how patients make decisions about taking anti-psychotic medication. Within the literature a range of factors that influence compliance in people with schizophrenia have been identified.

Given these limitations, what factors influence compliance in people with schizophrenia? Patients with a physical disorder who accept that they have an illness and perceive it as serious ('are insightful') tend to be more compliant (Haynes, 1976). This is consistent with the Health Belief Model, which hypothesises that individuals reach decisions on health actions based on their perception of the seriousness of the illness, their susceptibility to it and the benefits of adherence (Babiker, 1986). In studies of non-psychiatric patients this model generally shows a modest ability to predict/explain treatment compliance (Meichenbaum and Tusk, 1987). In schizophrenia, insight – defined as awareness of illness, an ability to recognise symptoms as part of an illness and acceptance of treatment – has also been associated with compliance. A number of studies examined the relationship between insight and compliance with generally consistent results, despite substantive differences in operational definitions of insight (Lin et al., 1979; Marder et al., 1983; Buchanan, 1992; Kemp and David, 1996).

A number of interpersonal factors (such as the therapist's ability to listen and empathise with the patient) and relationship factors (liking and trusting the therapist; the patient's level of involvement in treatment decisions including discussion of the patient's beliefs, concerns and expectations) have been shown to correlate with compliance in patients with physical disorders (Haynes, 1976). Patients' interactions with the therapist, including the process of formulating perceptions, therapist influence and the patient's evaluation of the treatment, are incorporated into the 'Theory of Reasoned Action' (Cochran and Gitlin, 1988). However, the ability of this model to explain or predict compliance has not been shown.

When asked, patients indicate that, subjectively, side-effects have a significant impact on compliance (Renton et al., 1963; Wieden et al., 1986). When this was examined more objectively, findings were equivocal and van Putten (1974) demonstrated an increased incidence of EPS in non-compliant patients. However, this finding has not been consistently replicated. In a two-year prospective study, Buchanan (1992) found no correlation between akathisia and compliance. Fleischhacker et al. (1994) also failed to establish a link between EPS and compliance in patients receiving long-term anti-psychotic treatment.

There is some evidence that a number of other factors may influence compliance: McEvoy et al. (1989) suggested that compliance was substantially higher in patients whose medication was supervised by a family member; Swofford et al. (1996) found that compliance rates were much lower in patients with a co-morbid substance misuse diagnosis. Other factors that are suggested within the literature as affecting compliance, but that lack any empirical evidence, include the complexity of treatment regimes (Parkin et al., 1976) and the patient's socio-cultural background (Piatkowska and Farnill, 1992).

Factors that enhance compliance

Adams and Howe (1993) examined factors that were likely to predict good compliance in 44 psychotic in-patients. The greater the number of indirect benefits of medication (i.e., 'keeps me out of hospital' or 'it allows me to make new friends'), the more compliant patients were. Similar results were reported by Chan (1984) who observed that compliant patients had generally derived positive benefits from medication.

Addressing insight, beliefs about treatment, side-effects and the other factors that influence compliance may improve compliance, and consequently the health, of people with schizophrenia.

Summary of reasons why patients do not comply

- Antipsychotic medication does not achieve its clinical potential.
- Fifty per cent of patients are non-compliant with medication.
- Factors that affect compliance include patients' awareness of their illness, their beliefs about treatment, the side-effects they experience from medication and their use of non-prescribed substances.

Assessment of factors that affect compliance

As the previous section demonstrated, there is a high level of non-compliance with medication. Three specific issues were identified as being relevant: insight into their illness, beliefs about treatment and side-effects of anti-psychotic medication. Measures are available that allow these issues to be quantified in a way that is both valid and reliable, however. Consequently, careful assessment of these factors will provide an important basis from which interventions may develop to increase compliance.

Insight: expanded schedule for the assessment of insight (SAI-E; Kemp and David, 1997)

The expanded schedule for the assessment of insight is a 10-item clinician-rated scale. Items are rated on a three-point scale based on a mental state examination (such as the KGV – see below) and specific additional questions described in the measure. Scores are expressed as a percentage of total insight and satisfactory reliability and validity have been reported (Kemp and David, 1997).

Beliefs about treatment: Hogan drug attitude inventory (DAI-30; Hogan et al., 1983)

The Hogan drug attitude inventory (DAI-30) is a 30-item self-report measure predictive of compliance in people with schizophrenia and useful in eliciting patients' beliefs about treatment. Each statement is rated as being true or false. The measure produces a total score ranging from +30 to −30; a positive score predicting compliance and a negative score non-compliance. The scale has been shown to have a degree of discriminative validity, with 89% agreement between the DAI and clinician rating of whether patients were compliant or non-compliant.

Side-effects: Liverpool University neuroleptic side-effect rating scale (LUNSERS; Day et al., 1995)

The LUNSERS is a 51-item self-report measure of the side-effects of anti-psychotic medication. Forty-one items covering psychological, neurological, autonomic, hormonal and miscellaneous side-effects were constructed by rephrasing items from the UKU adverse events measure (Linjaerde et al., 1987) so that they could be self-rated. The remaining 10 items were 'red herrings', referring to symptoms which were not known anti-psychotic side-effects (e.g., hair loss). Each item is rated on a five-point scale ranging from 'not at all' to 'very much', based on how frequently the patient has experienced the side-effect in the last month. The LUNSERS is an efficient, reliable and valid method of monitoring anti-psychotic side-effects (Day et al., 1995).

Psychopathology: KGV (Krawiecka et al., 1977)

It may also be useful to more formally assess a patient's psychopathology to evaluate the effectiveness of pharmacotherapy. Clinically the most widely used measure of psychopathology is the KGV (Krawiecka et al., 1977), a standardised psychiatric assessment scale for rating chronic psychotic patients.

Interventions to enhance compliance

Given the relationship between good compliance and outcome it is perhaps surprising how little research effort has been devoted to devising and testing interventions to improve the taking of prescribed anti-psychotic medication. A range of interventions has been evaluated in patients with both physical and mental disorders, although much of the research has focused on schizophrenia or acute psychosis. The interventions that have been tested include patient education (Seltzer et al., 1980; Stricker et al., 1986; Smith et al., 1992; Macpherson et al., 1996a Gray, 2000), behavioural interventions (Boczkowski et al., 1985) and cognitive behavioural interventions (Hayward et al., 1995; Kemp et al., 1996, 1998). Although the number of patients in these studies was generally quite small, statistically significant increases in medication adherence were found following some of the interventions. On a cautionary note, however, very few of the trials reported the impact of the intervention on clinical outcomes and, because of the small sample sizes used in the studies, the possibility of a false-negative (type II) error is quite high.

Educational interventions

Educational interventions aim to provide information to patients about both their illness and medication with the goal of increasing understanding and promoting compliance.

Group educational interventions were tested by Stricker et al. (1986) and Smith et al. (1992). The curriculum for the Stricker et al. (1986) medication education groups was divided into two parts. The first part consisted of six, weekly, didactic presentations about the major drugs used in psychiatry, the risks associated with substance misuse and the biochemical theory of schizophrenia. During the second part, over a four-week period, weekly discussions took place about the importance of taking medication, communication with physicians, and the benefits of long-term medication adherence. The groups were large, with up to 15 patients attending each. Unfortunately, following the end of the groups no difference in compliance or attitudes towards treatment were observed. However, significant improvements in patients' knowledge were observed. Patients also reported a high degree of satisfaction with the intervention.

Smith et al. (1992) evaluated a group educational intervention based on material developed for family psycho-education (Smith and Birchwood, 1987). The concept, symptoms and treatment of schizophrenia, in addition to basic symptom management strategies, were discussed with small groups of patients (five to six per group) in four fortnightly sessions. A booklet supported the information presented in the groups. Findings were similar to those reported by Stricker et al. (1986), in that no significant improvement in patients' compliance or insight was observed, although there was an increase in knowledge about medication.

Both of these studies suggest that whilst educational interventions are effective in improving patients' knowledge they have little impact on compliance with medication. One explanation for this finding may be that group interventions are not the most effective method of providing patients with information about their treatment. This was pursued by Macpherson et al. (1996) and Gray (2000) who examined whether individual patient education was effective in improving compliance with medication.

The intervention devised by Macpherson et al. (1996) consisted of either one or three individual sessions of education about medication. All sessions were individually tailored around an information booklet that was derived from the psycho-education literature (Smith and Birchwood, 1987). Again, patient knowledge about medication improved, with three sessions of education producing the greatest improvements. As in the study by Stricker et al. (1986) and Smith et al. (1992), compliance did not improve. Finally, Gray (2000) also showed that three sessions of structured patient education had no effect on patients' insight into their illness or their attitudes towards treatment.

The evidence suggests that patients want, and like, being given information either on a one-to-one basis or in a group, and this enhances their understanding of treatment. However, simply telling patients the importance of taking medication to prevent relapse does not change behaviour.

Behavioural interventions

If improving patients' understanding about their medication does not improve adherence then interventions may need to address some of the other factors that influence compliance. Boczkowski et al. (1985) suggested that helping patients to tailor their medication so that it fitted in with their daily routine (i.e., simplifying the treatment regime) would be effective in enhancing compliance. Patients were also encouraged to link taking medication with specific routine behaviours (e.g., making breakfast, turning off the television at night). Patients were also given a calendar with a dated slip of paper for each dose of anti-psychotic medication. They were told to keep the calendar with the medication and to remove the appropriate strip when they took it. Compliance was significantly improved in patients who received behavioural tailoring, suggesting that some practical and simple interventions can be effective.

Cognitive behavioural interventions

While behavioural tailoring attempts to address some of the factors affecting compliance, patients' reasons for not taking their medication are diverse.

The use of cognitive behavioural interventions to involve patients in their treatment and to encourage them to examine the range of factors affecting compliance have been researched by Hayward et al. (1995) and Kemp et al. (1996, 1998).

Medication self-management (Hayward et al., 1995) was based on motivational interviewing and aimed to allow patients and clinicians to work collaboratively to examine medication issues. Although no improvements in compliance were found, there was sufficient interest in the potential of the intervention to develop it further into a more structured one.

Kemp et al. (1996, 1998) devised compliance therapy based on medication self-management and drawing from motivational interviewing and cognitive behavioural techniques. Key principles included working collaboratively, emphasising personal choice and responsibility, and focusing on patients' concerns about treatment. The intervention was divided into three phases, which acknowledges that readiness to change is on a continuum. Phase 1 deals with patients' experiences of treatment by helping them review their illness history. In phase 2 the common concerns about treatment are discussed and the good and the bad things about treatment are explored. Phase 3 deals with long-term prevention and strategies for avoiding relapse. The intervention was evaluated by a large-scale randomised controlled trial (Kemp et al., 1996, 1998). Compliance therapy significantly enhanced treatment adherence and resulted in improved community tenure.

Implications for practice

Non-compliance with anti-psychotic medication is clearly a major preventable cause of relapse in patients with psychotic disorders. The causes of non-compliance are unclear but the evidence does suggest that a number of factors have a role to play and that individuals' reasons for stopping medication are idiosyncratic. A range of different pragmatic interventions to enhance compliance have been tested. Patient education enhances knowledge and behavioural tailoring improves compliance. Compliance therapy principles and techniques also seem to be particularly effective.

Medication management practice in the British National Health Service

Standards 4 and 5 of the National Service Framework (NSF) for mental health (Department of Health, 1999) aim to ensure that people with severe mental illnesses receive care and treatment that has a sound empirical basis. Good medication management, as described above and including assessment with valid and reliable measures and the application of compliance therapy techniques, is clearly identified within the framework as being integral to achieving these standards.

Much of the care and treatment that people with schizophrenia receive is delivered by mental health nurses. The SNMAC (1999) report indicated that, if NSF standards are to be achieved, there is an urgent need to improve the medication management skills of mental health nurses through training and the development of evidence-based policies and guidelines.

As has already been discussed, part of good medication management is the rigorous assessment of psychopathology, side-effects and subjective factors such as beliefs about treatment and insight. Mental health nurses' practice, especially in the assessment of side-effects, has been explored. For example, in a small survey of CPNs practice, Bennett et al. (1995) observed that on average CPNs screened patients for only three or four of the possible side-effects they might experience and there was no evidence of assessment using techniques other than an unstructured self-report. Gray (1998b) observed that mental health nurses do not ask patients about certain side-effects, such as sexual dysfunction, that may have a substantial impact on patients' decisions about taking medication.

Examining the impact of using valid and reliable assessment tools on the detection of EPS, Wieden et al. (1986) demonstrated that clinicians trained in using such measures were significantly more accurate at detecting side-effects than clinicians in routine practice. A survey by Gray et al. (2001) compared the reported practice of mental health nurses who had and had not received psychosocial intervention (PSI) training. Nurses who had received PSI training were significantly more likely to report using recognised measures of side-effects than those who were not.

Medication management: chapter summary

Medication management is a core skill of acute mental health nursing. Non-compliance with medication is a major preventable cause of relapse. The reasons why people do not take their medication are complex. The evidence suggests that good medication should consist of the following:

- a collaborative approach to working with patients;
- use of valid and reliable assessment tools to measure psychopathology, anti-psychotic side-effects, attitudes towards treatment, insight and compliance;
- logical prescribing of anti-psychotic medication;
- effective management of anti-psychotic side-effects;

- giving patients information about their illness and treatment;
- tailoring medication regimes to suit the patient;
- use of compliance therapy techniques.

The SNMAC (1999) report recognises the need for developing nurses' skills in this area. However, to improve practice throughout the British NHS, and to move towards achieving the standards set within the NSF, training on these will also need to be provided.

Annotated readings

Bazire, S. (2001) *Psychotropic Drug Directory 2001*. Wiltshire: Quay Books.

Very useful information about psychotropic drugs. A must-have book, updated annually.

Day, J.C., Wood, G., Dewey, M. and Bentall, R.P. (1995) 'A self-rating scale for measuring neuroleptic side-effects. Validation in a group of schizophrenic patients', *British Journal of Psychiatry*, 166: 650–3.

Information about the LUNSERS.

Gournay, K. and Gray, R. (2001) *Should Mental Health Nurses Prescribe?* London: Maudsley Publications.

A discussion on mental health nurse prescribing. Copies are available from Sarah Smith, Division of Psychological Medicine, Institute of Psychiatry, De Crespigny Park, London SE5 8AF.

Gray, R. (1999) 'Antipsychotics, side-effects and effective management', *Mental Health Practice*, 2 (7): 14–20.

Some useful strategies for managing anti-psychotic side-effects.

Haynes, R.B. Montague, P., Oliver, T. et al. (1999) *Interventions for Helping Patients Follow Prescriptions for Medication (Cochrane Review)*. In: The Cochrane Library, Issue 4, Oxford: Update Software.

Systematic review of compliance interventions.

Kemp, R., Hayward, P., Applewhaite, G. et al. (1996) 'Compliance therapy in psychoatic patients. Randomised controlled trial', *British Medical Journal*, 312: 345–9.

Kemp, R., Kirov, G., Everitt, P. et al. (1998) 'Randomised controlled trial of compliance therapy. 18-month follow-up', *British Journal of Psychiatry*, 172: 413–19.

The compliance therapy trials.

Macpherson, R., Jerrom, B. and Hughes, A. (1996) 'A controlled study of education about drug treatment in schizophrenia', *British Journal of Psychiatry*, 168: 709–17.

Patient education trial.

Resource section

Institute of Psychiatry website: **www.iop.kcl.ac.uk**

Useful information and links to other websites.

Compliance therapy manual
Kemp, R., Hayward, P., David, A., (1997) *Compliance Therapy Manual.* London: Bethlem and Maudsley NHS Trust.

Self-explanatory.

Maudsley prescribing guidelines
Taylor, D., McConnell, D., McConnell, H. et al. (1999) *The Bethlem and Maudsley NHS Trust Prescribing Guidelines*, 5th edn. London: Martin Dunitz.

Widely used prescribing guidelines.

South London and Maudsley NHS Trust drug information line: 020 7919 2999.

If you have a question and no one knows the answer, call this number and they will do their best to help.

Source of medication management training materials
Dr Richard Gray, Health Services Research Department, Institute of Psychiatry, De Crespigny Park, London SE5 8AF
E-mail: R.Gray@iop.kcl.ac.uk

Information on the KGV
Stuart Lancashire, Health Services Research Department, Institute of Psychiatry, De Crespigny Park, London SE5 8AF
E-mail: S.Lancashire@iop.kcl.ac.uk

KGV training videotapes
Keith Coupland, Brownhill Centre, Swindon Road, Cheltenham GL51 9EZ
E-mail: Keith@furlong.demon.co.uk

References

Adams, S.G. and Howe, J.T. (1993) 'Predicting medication compliance in a psychotic population', *Journal of Nervous and Mental Disease*, 181 (9): 558–60.
Babiker, I.E. (1986) 'Non-compliance in schizophrenia', *Psychiatric Developments*, 4: 329–337.

Bennett, J., Done, J. and Hunt, B. (1995) 'Assessing the side-effects of antipsychotic drugs: a survey of CPN practice', *Journal of Psychiatric and Mental Health Nursing*, 2 (3): 315–30.

Bigliani, V., Mulligan, R.S. and Acton, P.D. (1998) 'Preliminary results: D_2/D_3 like receptor binding in temporal cortex and striatum in sertindole and olanzapine treated patients', *Journal of Nuclear Medicine*, 39: 319.

Bleuler, M. (1974) 'The long-term course of schizophrenic psychoses', *Psychological Medicine*, 4: 244–54.

Boczkowski, J.A., Zeichner, A. and De Santo, N. (1985) 'Neuroleptic compliance among chronic schizophrenic outpatients: an intervention outcome report', *Journal of Consulting and Clinical Psychology*, 53: 666–71.

Buchanan, A. (1992) 'A two-year prospective study of treatment compliance in patients with schizophrenia', *Psychological Medicine*, 22: 787–97.

Chan, D.W. (1984) 'Medication compliance in a Chinese psychiatric outpatient setting', *British Journal of Medical Psychology*, 57: 81–9.

Churchill, D.N. (1985) 'Compliance: how to measure it', *Medicine of Canada*, 40: 1068–70.

Ciompi, L. (1980) 'Catamnestic long-term study of the course of life and ageing in schizophrenics', *Schizophrenia Bulletin*, 6: 606–18.

Claghorn, J., Chapman, J.P. and Abuzzahab, F.S. (1987) 'The risks and benefits of clozapine versus chlorpromazine', *Journal of Clinical Psychopharmacology*, 7: 377–84.

Cochran, S.D. and Gitlin, M.J. (1988) 'Attitudinal correlates of lithium compliance in bipolar affective disorders', *Journal of Nervous and Mental Disorders*, 176: 457–64.

Cramer, J.A. and Rosenheck, R. (1998) 'Compliance with medication regimens for mental and physical disorders', *Psychiatric Services*, 49: 196–201.

Creese, I., Burt, D.R. and Snyder, S.H. (1976) 'Dopamine receptor binding predicts clinical and pharmacological potencies of antipsychotic drugs', *Science*, 192: 481–3.

Day, J.C., Wood, G., Dewey, M. and Bentall, R.P. (1995) 'A self-rating scale for measuring neuroleptic side-effects. Validation in a group of schizophrenic patients', *British Journal of Psychiatry*, 166: 650–3.

Department of Health (1999) *The National Service Framework for Mental Health*. London: The Stationery Office.

Farde, L., Nordstrom, A.L. and Nyberg, S. (1992) D_1-, D_2 and 5-HT2-receptor occupancy in clozapine treated patients', *Journal of Clinical Psychiatry*, 55 (Supplement B): 67–9.

Flieschhacker, W.W., Meise, U., Günther, V. and Kurz, M. (1994) 'Compliance with antipsychotic drug treatment: influence of side-effects', *Acta Psychiatrica Scandinavica*, 382: 11–15.

Gabel, W. and Piezcker, A. (1985) 'One-year outcome of schizophrenic patients – the interaction of chronic and neuroleptic treatment', *Psychopharmacology*, 18: 235–9.

Gray, R. (1998a) 'Effective dosing in the use of antipsychotics for treatment of acute schizophrenia', *Mental Health Care*, 1 (9): 303–4.

Gray, R. (1998b) 'Primary care of schizophrenia: what are the roles of practice and community psychiatric nurses?', *Community Mental Health*, 1 (4): 5–7.

Gray, R. (1999) 'Antipsychotics, side-effects and effective management', *Mental Health Practice*, 2 (7): 14–20.

Gray, R. (2000) 'Does patient education enhance compliance with clozapine? A preliminary investigation', *Journal of Psychiatric and Mental Health Nursing*, 7: 285–6.

Gray, R., Wykes, T. and Parr, A.M. (2001) 'The use of outcome measures to evaluate the efficacy and tolerability of antipsychotic medication: a comparison of Thorn graduate and CPN practice', *Journal of Psychiatric and Mental Health Nursing*, 8: 191–6.

Haynes, R.B. (1976) 'A critical review of the "determinant" of patients' compliance with therapeutic regimens', in D.L. Sackett and R.B. Haynes, (eds), *Compliance with Therapeutic Regimens*. Baltimore: Johns Hopkins University Press.

Hayward, P., Chan, N. and Kemp, R. (1995) 'Medication self-management: a preliminary report of an intervention to improve medication compliance', *Journal of Mental Health*, 4: 511–17.

Helgason, L. (1990) 'Twenty year follow-up of first psychiatric presentation for schizophrenia: what could have been prevented?', *Acta Psychiatrica Scandinavica*, 81: 231–5.

Hogan, T.P., Awad, A.G. and Eastwood, R. (1983) 'A self-report scale predictive of drug compliance in schizophrenics: reliability and discriminative validity', *Psychological Medicine*, 13: 177–83.

Kane, J.M. (1989) 'Management strategies for the treatment of schizophrenia', *Journal of Clinical Psychiatry*, 60 (Supplement 12): 13–17.

Kane, J., Honigfeld, G., Singer, J. and Meltzer, H. (1988) 'Clozapine for the treatment-resistant schizophrenic. A double-blind comparison with chlorpromazine', *Archives of General Psychiatry*, 45: 789–96.

Kapur, S. and Remington, G. (1996) 'Serotonin–dopamine D_2 receptor occupancy with low dose haloperidol treatment: a PET study', *American Journal of Psychiatry*, 153: 466–73.

Kemp, R. and David, A. (1996) 'Psychosis: insight and compliance', *Current Opinion in Psychiatry*, 8 (6): 357–61.

Kemp, R. and David, A. (1997) 'Reasoning and delusions', *British Journal of Psychiatry*, 170: 398–405.

Kemp, R., Hayward, P., Applewhaite, G., Everitt, B., and David, A. (1996) 'Compliance therapy in psychoatic patients. Randomised controlled trial', *British Medical Journal*, 312: 345–9.

Kemp, R., Hayward, P. and David, A. (1997) *Compliance Therapy Manual*. London: Bethlem and Maudsley NHS Trust.

Kemp, R., Kirov, G., Everitt, B., Hayward, P. and David, A. (1998) 'Randomised controlled trial of compliance therapy: 18-month follow-up', *British Journal of Psychiatry*, 172: 413–19.

Kisling, W. (1994) 'Compliance, quality assurance and standards for relapse prevention in schizophrenia', *Acta Psychiatrica Scandinavica*, 89 (Supplement 382): 16–24.

Krawiecka, M., Goldberg, D. and Vaughn, M. (1977) 'A standardised psychiatric assessment scale for rating chronic psychotic patients', *Acta Psychiatrica Scandinavica*, 55: 299–308.

Lin, H.F., Spiga, R. and Fortsch, W. (1979) 'Insight and adherence to medication in chronic schizophrenics', *Journal of Clinical Psychiatry*, 40: 430–2.

Linjaerde, O., Ahlfors, U.G., Bech, P., Dencker, S.J. and Elgen, K. (1987) 'The UKU side-effects rating scale', *Acta Psychiatrica Scandinavica*, 76 (Supplement 334): 83–94.

McEvoy, J.P., Apperson, L.J. and Applebaum, P.S. (1989) 'Insight in schizophrenia. Its relationship to acute psychopathology', *Journal of Nervous and Mental Disease*, 177: 43–7.

Macpherson, R., Jerrom, B. and Hughes, A. (1996) 'A controlled study of education about drug treatment in schizophrenia', *British Journal of Psychiatry*, 168: 709–17.

Marder, S.R. (1999) 'Antipsychotic drugs and relapse prevention', *Schizophrenia Research*, 35 (Supplement): S87–S92.

Marder, S.R., Mebane, A., Chiem, C. et al. (1983) 'A comparison of patients who refuse and consent to neuroleptic treatment', *American Journal of Psychiatry*, 140: 470–2.

Matted, J.A. (1989) 'Clozapine for refractory schizophrenia: an open study of 14 patients treated for up to two years', *Journal of Clinical Psychiatry*, 50 (38I): 379–91.

Meichenbaum, D. and Tusk, D.C. (1987) *Facilitating Treatment Adherence: A Practitioner's Guidebook.* New York: Plenum Press.

Meltzer, H.Y., Bastani, B., Kwon, K.Y. and Sharpe, J. (1989) 'A prospective study of clozapine in treatment-resistant schizophrenic patients I: preliminary report', *Psychopharmacology*, 99: 68–72.

Moore, S. (1999) 'Behavioural pharmacology of the new generation of antipsychotic agents', *British Journal of Psychiatry*, 174 (Supplement 38): 5–11.

Parkin, D.M., Henney, C.R., Quirk, J., and Crooks, J. (1976) 'Deviation from prescribed drug treatment after discharge from hospital', *British Medical Journal*, 2 (6037): 686–8.

Piatkowska, O. and Farnill, D. (1992) 'Medication – compliance or alliance? A client-centred approach to increasing adherence', in D.J. Kavanagh (ed.), *Schizophrenia: An Overview and Practical Handbook*. London: Chapman and Hall.

Pilowsky, L.S., Costa, D.C., Ell, P.J., Murray, R.M., Verkoeff, N.P., and Kerwin, R.W. (1992) 'Clozapine, single photon emission tomography and the D_2 dopamine receptor blockade hypothesis of schizophrenia', *Lancet*, 340: 199–202.

Pilowsky, L.S., Costa, D.C., Ell, P.J., Murray, R.M., Verkoeff, N.P. and Kerwin, R.W. (1993) 'Antipsychotic medication D_2 dopamine blockade receptor blockade and clinical response: a 123I IBZM SPET single photon emission tomography study', *Psychological Medicine*, 23: 791–7.

Quitkin, F., Rifkin, A., Kane, J.M. and Klein, D.F. (1978) 'Long action versus injectable antipsychotics drugs in schizophrenics. A one year double-blind comparison in multiple episode schizophrenics', *Archives of General Psychiatry*, 35: 889–92.

Renton, C.A., Affleck, J.W. and Carstairs, G.M. (1963) 'A follow-up of schizophrenic patients in Edinburgh', *Acta Psychiatrica Scandinavica*, 39: 548–600.

Seltzer, A., Roncari, I. and Garfinkel, P. (1980) 'Effect of patient education on medication compliance', *Canadian Journal of Psychiatry*, 25: 638–45.

Shepherd, M., Watt, D. and Falloon, I. (1989) 'The natural history of schizophrenia: a five year follow-up study of outcome and prediction in a representative sample of schizophrenics', *Psychological Medical Monograph Supplement*, 15: 1–46.

Smith, J. and Birchwood, M. (1987) 'Relatives and patients as partners in the management of schizophrenia', *British Journal of Psychiatry*, 156: 654–660.

Smith, J., Birchwood, M. and Haddrell, A. (1992) 'Informing people with schizophrenia about their illness: the effect of residual symptoms', *Journal of Mental Health*, 1: 61–70.

Standing Nursing and Midwifery Advisory Committee (SNMAC) (1999) *Mental Health Nursing: Addressing Acute Concerns*. London: The Stationery Office.

Stricker, S.K., Amdur, M. and Dincin, J. (1986) 'Educating patients about psychiatric medication, failure to enhance compliance', *Psychosocial Rehabilitation*, 4: 15–28.

Swofford, C.D., Kasckow, J.W., Scheller-Gilkey, G. and Inderbitzen, L.B. (1996) 'Substance use: a powerful predictor of relapse in schizophrenia', *Schizophrenia Research*, 20: 145–51.

Taylor, D., McConnell, D. and McConnell, H. (2001) *The Bethlem and Maudsley NHS Trust Prescribing Guidelines*, 6th edn. London: Martin Dunitz.

van Putten, T. (1974) 'Why do schizophrenic patients refuse to take their medication?', *Archives of General Psychiatry*, 31: 67–72.

Wieden, P.J., Shaw, E. and Mann, J. (1986) 'Causes of neuroleptic non-compliance', *Psychiatric Annals*, 16: 571–8.

Wolff, R.J. and Colacino, D.M. (1961) 'A preliminary report on the continued post-hospital use of tranquillising drugs', *American Journal of Psychiatry*, 118: 499–503.

World Health Organisation (WHO) (1992) *The ICD-10 Classification of Mental and Behavioural Disorder*. Geneva: World Health Organisation.

Index